SpringerBriefs in Bioengineering

SpringerBriefs present concise summaries of cutting-edge research and practical applications across a wide spectrum of fields. Featuring compact volumes of 50 to 125 pages, the series covers a range of content from professional to academic. Typical topics might include: A timely report of state-of-the art analytical techniques, a bridge between new research results, as published in journal articles, and a contextual literature review, a snapshot of a hot or emerging topic, an in-depth case study, a presentation of core concepts that students must understand in order to make independent contributions.

More information about this series at http://www.springer.com/series/10280

Ali Cinar · Kamuran Turksoy

Advances in Artificial Pancreas Systems

Adaptive and Multivariable Predictive Control

Springer

Ali Cinar
Department of Biological
and Chemical Engineering
Illinois Institute of Technology
Chicago, IL
USA

Kamuran Turksoy
Department of Biomedical Engineering
Illinois Institute of Technology
Chicago, IL
USA

ISSN 2193-097X ISSN 2193-0988 (electronic)
SpringerBriefs in Bioengineering
ISBN 978-3-319-72244-3 ISBN 978-3-319-72245-0 (eBook)
https://doi.org/10.1007/978-3-319-72245-0

Library of Congress Control Number: 2018930365

Printed on acid-free paper

This Springer imprint is published by Springer Nature
The registered company is Springer International Publishing AG
The registered company address is: Gewerbestrasse 11, 6330 Cham, Switzerland

To Mine, Bedirhan and Melik (A. Cinar)
To Shadan and Naz (K. Turksoy)
for their love, support and inspiration.

Preface

Significant progress has been made in finding a *cure* for diabetes. Research in islet transplantation, islet growth from adult stem cells, and gene-based therapies shows good promise and will provide alternatives to cure diabetes. Advances in the *treatment* of diabetes have offered new technologies that ease the daily burden of people with diabetes, improve their quality of life, and extend their life span. They provide valuable technologies to reduce the impact of diabetes while waiting for a cure. The complexity of glucose homeostasis and the current level of technology challenge tight blood glucose concentration (BGC) regulation. Artificial pancreas (AP) systems that closely mimic the glucose-regulating function of a healthy pancreas automate BGC management, dramatically reducing diabetes-related risks and improving lives of people who have the disease. These systems will monitor glucose levels around the clock and automatically infuse the optimal amount of insulin, and potentially other BGC-stabilizing hormones, in a timely manner. The nonlinearities and time-varying changes of blood glucose dynamics, the occurrence of nonstationary disturbances, time-varying delays on measurements and insulin infusion, and noisy data from sensors provide challenges for the AP. Several different types of AP system designs have been proposed in recent years. Most systems rely exclusively on continuous glucose measurements and adjust the insulin infusion rate of a pump. Advances in wearable devices that report physiological data in real time enabled the use of additional information and the development of multivariable AP systems. Progress in long-term stable glucagon research enabled the development of dual-hormone AP system designs. Advances in smartphones and communications technologies, and in control theory contributed to the development of powerful control algorithms that can be executed on smartphones and computational capabilities installed in insulin pump systems. Techniques in system monitoring and supervision, fault detection and diagnosis, and performance assessment enabled advanced diagnostics and fault-tolerant control technologies for AP systems.

The goal of this book is to introduce recent developments and directions for future progress in AP systems. The material covered represents a culmination of several years of theoretical and applied research carried out by the authors and many prominent research groups around the world. The book starts with some historical background on diabetes and AP systems. The heart of the AP system—sophisticated algorithms that function on a smartphone or similar device—collects information from the sensor of a continuous glucose monitor and wearable devices, computes the optimal insulin dose to infuse, and instructs the insulin pump to deliver it. The early chapters of the book provide information about currently available devices, techniques, and algorithms to develop AP systems. Then, several factors such as meals, exercise, stress and sleep (MESS) that challenge AP systems are discussed. In later chapters, both empirical (data-driven) and first-principles-based modeling techniques are presented. Recursive modeling techniques that enable adaptive control of the AP are introduced and integrated with multiple-input models used in adaptive control. Different control strategies such as model predictive, proportional–integral–derivative, generalized predictive, and fuzzy logic control are introduced. Physiological variables that can provide additional information to enable feedforward action to deal with MESS challenges are proposed. Several additional modules to address the challenges of MESS factors are discussed, and a multimodule adaptive multivariable AP system is described. Fault detection and reconciliation of missing or erroneous data and assessment of controller performance are presented to develop modules for fault-tolerant operation of an AP. A summary of recent clinical studies is provided, and the directions of future developments are discussed. Over 300 references are listed to provide a database of publications in many AP-related areas.

Progress in AP research is fueled by the passion of the researchers, advances in many technologies, and visionary leadership from federal agencies (National Institute of Diabetes and Digestive and Kidney Diseases (NIDDK) and its Diabetes Technology Program) and foundations (Juvenile Diabetes Research Foundation (JDRF) and Helmsley Charitable Trust). All academic research groups and industry have benefited from the fertile environment created during the past decade to advance the AP technology.

The authors are grateful to the members of the Cinar lab who participated in artificial pancreas research over the years (Dr. Meriyan Eren-Oruklu, Dr. Elif Seyma Bayrak, Jianyuan Feng, Sediqeh Samadi, Iman Hajizadeh, Mert Sevil, Colleen Monforti, Nicole Frantz, Rachel Brandt, Dr. Xia Yu, Caterina Lazaro, Zacharie Maloney, Dr. Mudassir Rashid) and to our collaborators in clinical studies at the University of Chicago (Dr. Elizabeth Littlejohn), University of Illinois at Chicago (Dr. Laurie Quinn, Dr. Lisa Sharp), and York University (Dr. Michael Riddell). The financial support provided by NIDDK (1DP3DK101077 and 1DP3DK101075), JDRF (17-2013-472, 3-PDF-2016-175-A-N, and 1-INO-2015-137-A-N), and by the University of Chicago Diabetes Research and Training Center (DRTC) funded by NIDDKP30DK020595 is gratefully acknowledged.

We hope that the AP technologies presented in this book will excite many researchers to address various challenges in managing diabetes and contribute to the development of the next-generation AP systems.

Chicago, IL, USA
September 2017

Ali Cinar
Kamuran Turksoy

Contents

Abbreviations

ACCM	Accelerometer
AP	Artificial pancreas
AR	Autoregressive
ARMA	Autoregressive moving average
ARMAX	Autoregressive moving average with exogenous inputs
BGC	Blood glucose concentration
CGM	Continuous glucose monitoring
CHO	Carbohydrates
CSII	Continuous subcutaneous insulin infusion
DG4P	Dexcom G4 Platinum
DG5M	Dexcom G5 Mobile
DSP	Dexcom 7 Plus
MDII	Multiple daily insulin injections
MESS	Meals, exercise, sleep and stress
FDA	Food and Drug Administration
FL	FreeStyle Libre
FLR	Fuzzy logic rules
FN	FreeStyle Navigator
FNII	FreeStyle Navigator II
GPC	Generalized predictive control
HEA	Hypoglycemia early alarm system
HRM	Heart rate monitor
IOB	Insulin on board
IVGTT	Intravenous glucose tolerance test
JDRF	Juvenile Diabetes Research Foundation
MARD	Mean absolute relative difference
MIMO	Multi-input multi-output
MM	Minimal model
MPC	Model predictive control
PID	Proportional–integral–derivative

Ra	Rate of glucose appearance
Rd	Rate of glucose disappearance
RLS	Recursive least squares
RNN	Recurrent neural network
SAP	Sensor-augmented pump
SMBG	Self-monitoring of blood glucose
SISO	Single-input single-output
SVR	Support vector regression
T1D	Type 1 diabetes
T2D	Type 2 diabetes

Chapter 1
Introduction

Abstract A brief history of diabetes and artificial pancreas systems is presented. Diabetes is a metabolic disease where production and/or utilization of insulin is impaired, leading to elevated blood glucose levels. Blood glucose is the main source of energy for the human body. Insulin, a hormone made by the body, enables the glucose in the bloodstream to get into cells. Over time, elevated glucose levels leads to problems related to heart disease, stroke, kidney, eye, nerve, dental and foot. Diabetes has no cure yet, but advances in technology have improved treatment to manage the disease and keep blood glucose levels in the desired range. People with type 1 diabetes (no insulin production by the body) administer three to five insulin injections daily or infuse insulin with an insulin pump to regulate their blood glucose concentration. This manual regulation is laborious and many people still experience dangerous low and high glucose levels during their daily lives. An artificial pancreas automates insulin pumps by using a closed-loop controller that receives information from glucose sensors, and manipulates the infusion rate of the pump. This new technology has been under development over the last three decades to develop artificial pancreas systems that are safe and effective in glucose level management in people with diabetes under free living conditions.

Keywords Diabetes · History of diabetes · Artificial pancreas

1.1 Diabetes

Diabetes mellitus is a metabolic disorder with multiple etiologies. It is characterized by chronic hyperglycemia in response to ingestion of carbohydrates, fat, and protein, resulting from defects of insulin secretion, insulin action, or both (Alberti and Zimmet 1998). In 1964, the first World Health Organization (WHO) Expert Committee on diabetes mellitus classified the disorder as juvenile-onset and maturity-onset disease based on the patient's age (World Health Organization 1964). In 1980, a second

A. Cinar and K. Turksoy, *Advances in Artificial Pancreas Systems*,
SpringerBriefs in Bioengineering, https://doi.org/10.1007/978-3-319-72245-0_1

WHO Expert Committee changed the two groups of diabetes mellitus to insulin-dependent diabetes mellitus (IDDM) and noninsulin-dependent diabetes mellitus (NIDDM) (World Health Organization 1980). In 1999, WHO and American Diabetes Association (ADA) relabeled the groups as type 1 diabetes (T1D) and type 2 diabetes (T2D) (WHO Consultation 1999). The pancreases of people with T1D do not produce and secrete insulin, and insulin analogs must be administered from external sources. People with T2D have some insulin production, which may not be sufficient to regulate blood glucose levels and their efficiency to use insulin may be compromised.

According to the International Diabetes Federation, currently 387 million people are affected by diabetes worldwide which is estimated to increase by 205 million people by 2035 (Diabetes atlas 2014). Diabetes has been reported as the seventh leading cause of death in the USA, and the cost of diabetes has been estimated to be $174 billion in the USA in 2007 (Centers for Disease Control and Prevention 2011) and $612 billion worldwide in 2014 (Diabetes atlas 2014). Every seven seconds one person dies from diabetes or its complications worldwide (Diabetes atlas 2014). In the USA, heart disease was noted to be the cause of 68% and stroke 16% of diabetes-related deaths in 2004. In 2005–2008, 67% of adults aged 20 years or older with self-reported diabetes had blood pressure greater than or equal to 140/90 millimeters of mercury (mm Hg) or used prescription medications for hypertension. Diabetes is the leading cause of new cases of blindness. About 44% of all new cases of kidney failure was attributed to diabetes in 2008. About 60–70% of people with diabetes have mild-to-severe forms of nervous system damage. More than 60% of nontraumatic lower-limb amputations occur in people with diabetes (Centers for Disease Control and Prevention 2011). In the USA, 5% of diabetes cases are T1D and approximately 85% of people living with T1D are adults (Prime Group for JDRF 2011).

1.2 History of Diabetes

Diabetes was described for the first time in an Egyptian papyrus (The Ebers papyrus) dating from c. 1550 BC where "too great emptying of the urine" is mentioned (Poretsky 2010; Polonsky 2012; Wikipedia 2017). Indian physicians identified and named the disease "honey urine" around the same period (Poretsky 2010). The name "diabetes" comes from the Greek word for the syphon (to pass through) for frequent and excessive urination. The adjective "mellitus" (honeyed) was added in the late eighteenth century (Rollo 1797). Several sources provide information about the history of diabetes and discovery of insulin from the ancient time to date (Poretsky 2010; Polonsky 2012; Wikipedia 2017; Holt et al. 2011). Early in the twentieth century, several researchers had suggested that diabetes resulted from a lack of a hormone secreted by the islets of Langerhans in the pancreas which was named "insulin" (Michael 1982). The challenge was to find a way to extract insulin from the pancreas before it was destroyed in order to conduct experimental studies with it (Bliss 2013). This was achieved in 1920, and insulin was extracted from dogs and later from fetal calves (Michael 1982). Experiments on dogs confirmed the role of insulin in regulating the blood glucose concentration (BGC) and treatment of human with T1D by insulin injection began. Various approaches for injecting insulin were developed over the years leading to insulin pens and insulin pumps. BGC measurement techniques progressed over time as well, to glucose meters that analyze BGC from a single drop of blood collected from finger tips and later to continuous glucose monitoring (CGM) systems. The availability of CGMs and insulin pumps enabled the development of AP systems for use under free-living conditions.

A watershed event in the automation of insulin delivery is the first hybrid AP system, the MiniMed 670G by Medtronic, approved by the U.S. FDA for prescription to people with T1D in 2017 (Medtronic 2017). The 670G is called a hybrid closed-loop AP that needs manual meal and exercise information. Additional research is needed to develop a fully automated AP that can function without any manual information and accommodate major disturbances to the BGC, such as meals, physical activity (exercise), sleep, and psychological stress (MESS). The critical importance of the commercial introduction of automated closed-loop control is the maturity of the AP technology that enabled the shift of responsibility and decision making from the individual with T1D to an automated algorithm for the first time.

1.3 Artificial Pancreas

In healthy subjects, BGC is regulated within tight limits (70–90 mg/dl of BGC) after overnight fasting conditions). The BGC range increases to 120–160 mg/dl following a meal depending on the meal size. The regulation of BGC to fasting levels is rapidly achieved (usually within 2–3 h). In people with T1D, BGC levels cannot be reduced to the normal range after a meal because of the lack of endogenous insulin, and BGC may increase up to 300–400 mg/dl if exogenous insulin is not administered. Similarly, fasting BGC can be as high as 150–250 mg/dl for untreated patients with T1D. Excess glucose in the blood can damage the blood vessels, leading to several complications such as cardiovascular disease, damage to kidneys, nerves, and eyes, and difficulty in wound healing.

People with T1D need to administer multiple daily insulin injections (MDII) (3–5 per day and usually pre-meal) or use insulin pumps for continuous subcutaneous insulin injection (CSII). In CSII, basal insulin is infused continuously and bolus insulin in administered before meals to maintain BGC in the target range (70–180 mg/dl). People with T1D may experience hypoglycemia (BGC$\leq$ 70 mg/dl) episodes that may be caused by insulin doses that are too large in relation to the BGC, reduced food intake, extensive physical activity, or slow absorption of currently available "fast-acting" insulins. Hypoglycemia causes dizziness, unconsciousness, seizures and if untreated, diabetic coma or death. Fear of hypoglycemia is prevalent among patients with T1D and a concern in use of insulin pumps. The success rate of maintaining BGC in normal range by manual injection therapies has been limited. Changing life style, and occurence of psychological stress (acute and chronic), illness, and

Fig. 1.1 Artificial pancreas

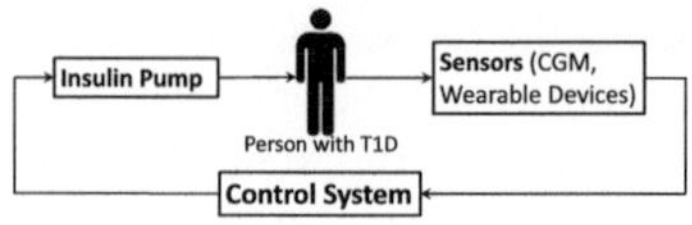

physical activity are some of the factors that affect the effectiveness of insulin and necessitate careful estimation of manual injection amounts.

An AP will automate insulin pump operation by using a closed-loop controller that receives information from sensors, computes the optimal insulin amount to be infused, and manipulates the infusion rate of the pump (Fig. 1.1). An AP that can predict BGC accurately and compute infusion rates that will keep BGC in the target range without causing hypoglycemia would be very beneficial. Control systems that minimize the information to be entered by the user to the AP such as meal and exercise information would make life easier for people with T1D.

The first clinical experiments of closed-loop BGC control systems date back to 1974 (Albisser et al. 1974) with intravenous sampling of BGC and intravenous feeding of dextrose to simulate food and insulin had remarkable success. The challenge of developing an AP for daily use was to find safe technologies for measurement of BGC and delivery of insulin. Glucose sensors of CGM systems that collect subcutaneous glucose concentration information and insulin pumps that deliver insulin to subcutaneous tissue were major contributors to the development of APs for use under free-living conditions. The advances in smartphones and communication technologies provided the critical mobile computing capability for developing AP systems. Today, microprocessors and memory installed inside insulin pump systems or smartphones enable the implementation of APs such as the Medtronic 670G and other AP technologies.

Advances in technology were complemented by strategic initiatives by the Juvenile Diabetes Research Foundation (JDRF) and the National Institute of Diabetes and Digestive and Kidney Diseases (NIDDK). JDRF initiated an artificial pancreas research consortium in 2006 and proposed a sequential road map to AP system development in 2009 that guided many AP research projects (Kowalski and Lum 2009). In the same period, the Diabetes Technology Program of the NIDDK provided significant investment to AP research. NIDDK, in collaboration with the FDA initiated public workshops to facilitate medical device innovation in the development of the AP (Klonoff et al. 2011). Two annual international conference series, Diabetes Technology Meeting (DTM) and Advanced Technologies and Treatments for Diabetes (ATTD), brought academic researchers, FDA and NIH representatives, and industry to provide a forum to report recent developments and discuss future research needs. The fertile research environment created by JDRF and NIDDK enabled many multidisciplinary teams to address various challenges ranging from the development of better glucose sensors and insulin pumps to novel model-based hypoglycemia prediction and automatic control algorithms. National and international collaborations accelerated R&D efforts and major advances have been made in hardware, information processing, decision making, and automatic control.

The JDRF Road Map was recently updated based on achievements in AP research and advances in technology since 2009, condensing AP development road map from the original six steps to three, and has bifurcated into automated insulin delivery approaches utilizing only insulin and multihormone approaches (insulin and glucagon, insulin and amylin, or insulin and other glucose-modulating agents) (Kowalski 2015).

Glucose–insulin dynamics in the human body has high levels of intra- and inter-person variability. The majority of the current AP systems rely on fixed physiological models. These models are developed based on measurements of complex physiological phenomena which requires detailed knowledge about the human body. However, due to variability of glucose–insulin dynamics of different people with T1D and variations in glucose dynamics of the same person depending on various conditions, these models cannot be fitted to every person with T1D. They must be re-defined/tuned for different patients. Real-time modification may also be required due to different conditions such as MESS which are known to have significant effects on glucose–insulin dynamics. The computation cost of fixed physiological models is also high due to nonlinearities and large number of equations. Various automatic control strategies with fixed physiological modeling have been investigated during the last three decades. The parameters of the control strategies should also be retuned when a patient's metabolism, physical activities, or emotional state changes significantly. Adaptive control with frequently updated models provide an attractive solution for finding representative models for use in model-based controllers that respond better to the current state of the user.

Many current-generation AP systems are not fully automated. Disturbances such as meals or exercise are manually announced to the AP system or the user makes changes to the operation of the AP before beginning an exercise. The problem of over/under estimation of carbohydrate amounts in a meal still exists which may cause hypo/hyperglycemia, respectively. Manually information announcement imposes extra burdens to parents who have children with T1D. They must do the calculation of carbohydrates in their meals and be careful of their physical activities. Next-generation APs are expected to be fully automated.

The current AP systems are developed based on only CGM measurements, with the exception of the multivariable AP developed by Cinar and co-workers (Turksoy et al. 2013b, 2014b). The effect of many factors such as exercise, sleep, or meal is seen in BGC with a time-varying delay. An additional delay caused by mass transfer limitations from the blood vessels to subcutaneous tissue is added when CGM measurements are used. An AP that is based only on CGM information cannot act fast enough to take action to minimize the possibility of exercise-induced hypoglycemia. By the time the effect is reported by CGM measurements, it might be too late for an AP system to manage glucose levels because the infused insulin may be delivered too late to balance the factors that caused the glucose increase. In addition to glucose measurement delays, insulin diffusion from the subcutaneous tissue to the blood stream has significant delay as well. For example, exercise at moderate levels increases insulin sensitivity which causes more glucose to be absorbed from the blood stream with the same amount of insulin. An AP system that is not aware of exercise may cause hypoglycemia due to lack of information about insulin sensitivity change. Additional data from wearable devices can be collected in real time to capture exercise information before BGC is affected and initiate actions to mitigate the effects of physical activity.

People with T1D may experience hypoglycemia episodes during their daily lives. The brain uses exclusively glucose for energy and when BGC drops, its functions are impaired. Their brain is not able to make rational decisions during severe hypoglycemia and implement measures to increase the BGC to safe levels. Many people with T1D state that they had very severe hypoglycemia (20–30 mg/dl) at least once in their life, such that, even when they knew that they must consume some carbohydrates they were not able to take action (Edelman 2007). Factors ranging from excessive overdosing of insulin to insufficient carbohydrate consumption, exercise, illness, and emotional stress may cause hypoglycemia. If hypoglycemia occurs during sleep, patients may not be aware of low glucose levels and may not wake up even when hypoglycemia alarms are issued. Fear of hypoglycemia is an important concern for people with T1D. Surveys indicate people with T1D have reduced fear of hypoglycemia if they use an AP system. Hence, AP system must have reliable algorithms for predicting hypoglycemia and regulating BGC by control action, rescue carbohydrates, and/or dual-hormone use.

The development of a fully automated AP that can function without any manual information and accommodate MESS will necessitate additional research to develop multivariable and adaptive AP systems that use information from wearable devices such as wristbands and modify their models used in model-predictive alarm and control systems to adapt to the changes in the metabolic state of the user.

Since the AP system uses several equipment such as sensors, transmitters, receivers, control units, and pumps, it is prone to equipment failures that can cause missing signals, outliers, and erroneous insulin delivery. For example, a sudden increase in CGM value due to sensor error may cause an AP to overdose insulin,

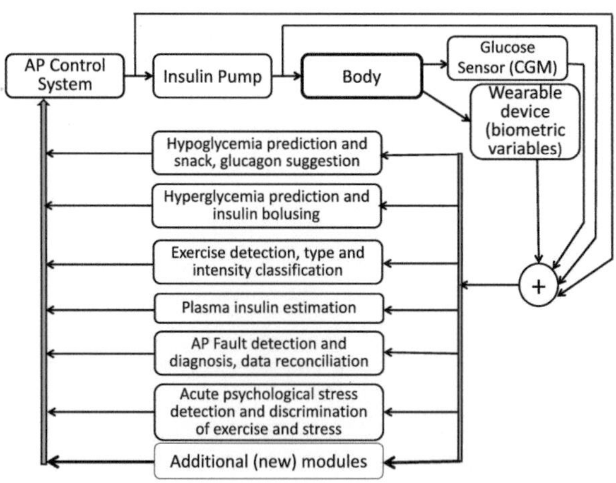

Fig. 1.2 Flowchart of a multivariable artificial pancreas with its modules

which may cause hypoglycemia. And a blockage in the infusion set or occlusion in the subcutaneous tissue may prevent insulin flow to the bloodstream and cause hyperglycemia. Hence, future AP systems must have a fault (failure) detection and diagnosis, and data reconciliation module that can monitor the AP system for possible equipment failures and implement fault-tolerant control and smooth transition to manual operation if needed.

The next-generation APs will have multiple modules that accommodate MESS challenges and provide fault-tolerant operation. The information flow and coordination of activities (Fig. 1.2) are more complex, and some functions of the AP may be executed in the pump system controller, others on a dedicated smartphone and on a server in the cloud depending on the intensity of computations and need to access large amounts of historical data. This distributed architecture must be implemented with proper safety and security features and reliable communications. Additional modules would include fault detection and diagnosis, data reconciliation, mitigation of sleep and psychological acute stress effects, controller performance assessment, and control system reconfiguration.

Chapter 2
Components of an Artificial Pancreas System

Abstract This chapter provides an extensive review of the components of artificial pancreas (AP) systems. Continuous glucose monitoring (CGM) sensors, insulin pumps and control algorithms are the three basic components of all AP systems. Information about currently available CGM sensors and insulin pumps is provided. Multivariable AP systems use information from wearable devices in addition to CGM information. Various wearable devices that can be used in an AP system are described. A brief description of control algorithms is also introduced. A more comprehensive discussion on control algorithms is provided in later chapters.

Keywords Continuous glucose monitoring sensors · Wearable sensors
Biometric variables · Insulin pumps · Control algorithms

All AP systems have three basic components: sensors, controllers, and insulin pumps. All APs that are being launched for consumer use (either commercially available or in pivotal clinical studies) rely on glucose sensors. A few research groups started experimenting with sensors that use heart rate and/or accelerometer information to detect exercise. The speed, accuracy, and reliability of subcutaneous glucose sensors are continuously improving, and the time periods that they can be used safely (as approved by the US FDA) are increasing. Alternative implantable glucose sensor technologies are maturing as well, to provide 90 days of continuous use as embedded sensors. Control systems range from proportional–integral–derivative (PID) controllers enriched by estimators to model predictive and adaptive controllers to knowledge-based systems with fuzzy logic. Insulin delivery pumps offered by various manufacturers have different features to provide freedom of choice to users. Some AP designs have included the controller in the pump system, while others prefer a smartphone to run the control system. A good account of the technologies available for closed-loop control of BGC until 2007 is given in a recent book (Chee and Fernando 2001).

A. Cinar and K. Turksoy, *Advances in Artificial Pancreas Systems*,
SpringerBriefs in Bioengineering, https://doi.org/10.1007/978-3-319-72245-0_2

2.1 Glucose Sensors

Currently, people with T1D use two primary methods in their daily lives to measure BGCs: capillary BGC measurements and CGM. Capillary BGC testing, also called self-monitoring of blood glucose (SMBG) (Vashist 2013), has been used for decades. It is fraught with variability and concern for accuracy in glucose meters compared to chemistry laboratory testing of blood samples because values reported by SMBG devices may be affected by meter calibration, ambient temperature, size and quality of sample drop of blood, high levels of interfering substances in the blood, hematocrit, humidity, and age of test strips (Ginsberg 2009). Patients can also generate additional clinically relevant BGC measurement errors such as residues of sugar-containing substances on fingers that cause a falsely high BGC or moist fingers that cause falsely low BGC (Downie 2013). The advantage of SMBG is to provide readings of BGC as opposed to CGM that provide glucose concentration in subcutaneous tissue.

CGM is a minimally invasive system with subcutaneous sensors to measure glucose levels in the interstitial fluid in real time (Vashist 2013; Klonoff 2005). When CGMs were first introduced, they had a sensor, a wireless transmitter, and a receiver with a display. Since many CGM users had insulin pumps as well, an alternative system emerged that placed the receiver in the pump and used the display of the pump. A more recent trend is to use a smartphone "app" to receive the CGM sensor data to a smartphone, do glucose level trend analysis and display various graphs to the user and broadcast the information to others who are given the permission by the user. Hence, the term CGM is also used to refer to the sensor and transmitter unit. There is a delay between BGC and glucose concentration in the interstitial fluid; hence, the values reported by the CGM trail BGC. The delay is estimated to be in the range of 3–12 min (Bequette 2010). This delay may not be important when CGMs are used to monitor glucose level variations, but if they are used in an AP, they affect its performance because delays in measured variable information influence the magnitude and timing of insulin infusion decisions.

Current CGMs require calibration with SMBG data at least twice per day. New generations of CGMs have been announced to extend their use to 14 days and reduce the number of daily calibrations to one, and then eliminate the need of daily calibrations by providing reliable factory calibrations. CGMs have 5-min sampling time to report glucose levels frequently. Observing the trends in glucose levels throughout the day rather than interpreting infrequent readings of BGC by SMBG empowers people with T1D and their care providers. It allows the patients to better understand their fasting and postprandial glucose trends and the effects of other factors such as physical activity on BGC. In SMBG, the patient may fail to recognize hypo- or hyperglycemic episodes if they are asymptomatic and do not happen to check their BGC at the time of the event (Vashist 2013). CGMs enable both the physician and patient to attempt to maintain physiologic glucose levels, adjust the insulin dose, and (most importantly) prevent dangerous glucose excursions, particularly hypoglycemia. CGM use can reduce hemoglobin A1C (a measure of average glucose control over the previous three months) and time spent in a hypoglycemic state, in both patient-led and physician-driven cohorts (Riveline et al. 2012). The JDRF CGM controlled randomized trial (Juvenile Diabetes Research Foundation Continuous Glucose Monitoring Study Group and Others 2008), the 2006 Guard Control Study (Deiss et al. 2006), and a recent study by OConnell et al. (2009) showed that adults with T1D who used CGM with SMBG had reduced A1C levels versus SMBG alone and were able to maintain glycemic control for 12 months without an increase in frequency of hypoglycemic excursions (Cengiz et al. 2011). However, there are conflicting data in the pediatric diabetic population, as a meta-analysis reported no significant difference between CGM versus SMBG in A1C reduction in T1D pediatric patients (Vashist 2013; Cengiz et al. 2011; Poolsup et al. 2013; Golicki et al. 2008), necessitating additional research to elucidate CGM effectiveness in the pediatric population. There are some disadvantages to the CGM: The insertion of a subcutaneous sensor may cause some discomfort, the sensor–transmitter takes up "real estate" space on the body of the user, and use of CGMs has higher cost (Klonoff 2005). Efforts to cover the cost of CGM use in retiree populations in the USA have increased in recent years.

Several CGMs are available today, including the systems by Medtronic, Dexcom, and Abbott (Vashist 2013). Many studies have examined CGMs and compared the reference glucose measurements to the corresponding CGM results by using the mean absolute relative deviation (MARD), a number that reports the average disparity between the sensor and capillary BGC readings obtained simultaneously. Lower MARD values indicate better CGM performance (Vashist 2013; Cengiz et al. 2011; Pleus et al. 2013). MARD is calculated both over the entire set of samples and in specific ranges such as hypo-, hyper-, and euglycemia. Some studies also consider the rate-of-change accuracy of the CGM, since reliable measurements during rapidly changing BGC episodes are critical.

Medtronic has the Enlite CGM that can be used for up to six days. The Enlite sensor is used in the USA in conjunction with the MiniMed 530G insulin pump. The Enlite sensor with the MiniMed 530G algorithm has a MARD of 13.6% (Rodbard 2016). Medtronic also has the Guardian Sensor 3 CGM used with the MiniMed 670G insulin pump, which can be utilized for up to 7 days. It has a MARD of 9.64% and is the only CGM sensor approved by FDA to control insulin dosing with the 670G hybrid closed-loop system. This system has the capability to automatically adjust basal insulin rate every 5 min to keep BGC in range. The Dexcom G4 Platinum (DG4P) and Dexcom G5 Mobile (DG5M) manufactured by Dexcom lasts up to 7 days, and the receiver has a 20-feet range to communicate with the transmitter. The DG4P and DG5M have an aggregate MARD of 13% and 9%, respectively, in adults (Vashist 2013; Rodbard 2016). The DG4P and DG5M are integrated with the Dexcom STUDIO and Dexcom CLARITY software, respectively, that allow the patient to review glucose trends. The DG5M is the first FDA-approved CGM to be used in real-time treatment decisions without a confirmatory SMBG value. The DG5M also has European approval to be used in this manner (Report 2016). The DG5M data can be sent directly from the transmitter to a compatible smart device, such as an iPhone or Android phone, or a standard receiver. The DG4P and DG5M feature a new system called *Share* that allows CGM data to be sent from the receiver via Bluetooth to a nearby iPhone, which if connected to the Internet allows for remote monitoring capabilities (Rodbard 2016; Dexcom 2016). Abbott developed the FreeStyle Navigator (FN), the FreeStyle Navigator II (FNII), and the FreeStyle Libre (FL) (Damiano et al. 2013). The FNII sensor measures glucose every 1 min and lasts up to 5 days (Vashist 2013). The FNII is a more compact device that provides glucose averages over 10 min. Its sensor can transmit data to the receiver within 30 meters and works during activities such as showering, swimming, and exercising (Vashist 2013). The FL sensor lasts up to 14 days. The FNII and FL have MARDs of 12.3% and 11.4%, respectively. The FNII has a built-in blood glucose meter that allows easier calibration. The FNII is not yet available in the USA as it is not yet approved by the FDA. The FL was recently approved by the FDA that can be used by adult (18 years of age and older) patients to make diabetes treatment decisions without calibration using an SMBG value. In a recent study, DG4P and FN had significantly lower MARD and significantly lower rate of very large errors than the Enlite and there were no significant difference between the DG4P and FN performance (Damiano et al. 2014). These CGMs are the successors of previous models such as the Dexcom 7 Plus and Medtronic Guardian that have been discontinued (Damiano et al. 2013). Since the first development of CGMs in the 2000s, sensor lifetime, accuracy, and frequency of required calibrations have all been significantly improved. As research progresses, newer generations of CGMs will provide more accurate data.

All CGMs in the market have alerts for high and low glucose levels and rapid changes in glucose levels (Vashist 2013). The user may miss the alarms. Responses to alarms are operator dependent, and users may ignore them. Current CGMs have addressed many challenges and reliability and accuracy (time delay) issues faced by previous generations of CGMs. For CGMs in early 2000s, 39% of CGM readings satisfied ADA precision criteria to be within ±10% of BGC from a SMBG, while 19% of readings satisfied the criteria to be within ±5% (Guerci et al. 2003). Current models have eliminated interference from acidominophen and vitamin C, increased reliability and transmission range, and improved MARD values. CGMs provide valuable information on glucose patterns, allowing people with diabetes to maintain glycemic control, lower their A1C levels, and avoid hypoglycemia (Vashist 2013; Klonoff 2005; Poolsup et al. 2013). Due to the reliance on SMBG for calibration, the latter remains a component of all APs until factory-calibrated CGMs for nonadjunctive use in treatment decisions become commercially available. Table 2.1 lists various subcutaneous glucose sensors.

An alternative class of glucose sensors are implantable sensors that are inserted under the skin by simple procedures that can be performed in a doctor's office (Senseonics 2017). They have longer periods of use (90 days or more), and they are better protected from physical damage. They exchange information with their transmitters and are powered by the transmitter via near-field communication. For example, Eversense by Senseonics has a use labeling of 90 days, and its next generation is announced to be 50% smaller with a 180-day life. A disadvantage is the need to insert and then remove the sensor with a surgical procedure at the end of its useful life. This procedure will become less frequent as their use life increases.

Table 2.1 Subcutaneous glucose sensors. Manufacturer listed in parentheses

Enlite Sensor with MiniMed 530G Pump: (Medtronic) Sensor life: 6 days, glucose sampling time: 5 min, MARD: 13.6%. It has remote monitoring capability and requires calibration every 12 h. Price for a one-month supply of sensors is $473, for the transmitter is $706, and for the pump is $7899. The system can connect to Apple devices with iOS 8 and 9 and Android devices with OS 5.0 and 6.0. It has FDA approval for use by patients 16 years and older who are not pregnant or on dialysis. The system provides predictive alerts up to 30 min in advance for high and low BG excursions, for excessive rates of change of BG, and for required calibrations of the sensor
Guardian Sensor 3 with MiniMed 670G Pump: (Medtronic) Sensor life: 7 days, glucose sampling time: 5 min, MARD: 9.64%. It does not have remote monitoring capability and requires calibration every 12 h. Price for a one-month supply of sensors is $475, for the transmitter is $706, and for the pump is $7899. It has FDA approval to control insulin dosing for patients 14 years and older who are not pregnant. The system provides predictive alerts up to 30 min in advance for high and low BG excursions and for excessive rise rates of BG
Dexcom G4 Platinum (DG4P): (Dexcom) Sensor life: 7 days, glucose sampling time: 5 min, MARD: 13%. It has remote monitoring capability and requires calibration every 12 h. Price for a pack of four sensors is $539, for the transmitter is $864, and for the receiver is $756. The Share app is compatible with iOS and watchOS software, and the Follow app is compatible with iOS and iWatchOS software as well as Android devices. The receiver sends glucose data to a smart device via Bluetooth. The system has FDA approval for use by patients 18 years and older who are not critically ill, pregnant, or on dialysis. It provides high and low BG excursion alerts and BG rise and fall rate alerts
Dexcom G5 Mobile (DG5M): (Dexcom) Sensor life: 6 days, glucose sampling time: 5 min, MARD: 9%. It has remote monitoring capability and requires calibration every 12 h. Price for a pack of 4 sensors is $539, for the transmitter is $864, and for the receiver is $756. The G5 Mobile app is compatible with iOS and watchOS software, and the Follow app is compatible with iOS and iWatchOS software and Android devices. Data can be sent directly from the transmitter via Bluetooth to a smart device, without a receiver. The system has FDA approval for use by patients 2 years and older who are not critically ill, pregnant, or on dialysis. It provides alerts for high and low BG excursions and BG rise and fall rate alerts
FreeStyle Navigator II (FNII): (Abbott) Sensor life: 5 days, glucose sampling time: 1 min, MARD: 12.3%. It does not have remote monitoring capability and requires calibration 1, 2, 10, 24, and 72 h post-sensor insertion. The system has USB connectivity for data upload to Mac or PC software. It does not have FDA approval. It is available in Europe for patients 6 years and older who are not pregnant or on dialysis. It provides audible and vibratory alerts for high and low BG excursions as well as projected BG excursions up to 30 min in advance
FreeStyle Libre (FL): (Abbott) Sensor life: 14 days, glucose sampling time: 1 min, MARD: 11.4%. The receiver requires a scan of the sensor to view the real-time glucose value and trend plus a line graph of the past 8 h of data. It has remote monitoring capability and does not require fingerstick calibration. The retail price for the sensor is $77 and for the receiver is $77. The system has USB connectivity for data upload to Mac or PC software. It has FDA approval for use in people 18 years of age and older with diabetes; after a 12-hour start-up period, it can be worn for up to 10 days (in the US). It is available in Europe for patients 4 years and older. The system does not provide automatic alerts
GlySens ICGM System: (GlySens) A fully implanted CGM sensor under development that is expected to have a lifetime of at least 1 year. It has FDA approval for investigational use only. Other proprietary information including its accuracy, compatibility, connectivity, and price is not yet available

(continued)

Table 2.1 (continued)

Eversense CGM system: (Senseonics) A fully implanted CGM sensor with a lifetime of 90 days. Glucose sampling time: 1 min, MARD: 11.4% in investigational studies. The system has remote monitoring capability; the smart transmitter connects directly to iOS and Android devices via Bluetooth without a separate receiver. It is currently in clinical studies for FDA approval. The system provides predictive on-body vibe alerts for high and low BG excursions

2.2 Sensors for Physiological (Biometric) Variables

Psychological chronic and acute stress, illness, and physical activity (physiological stress) can complicate BGC regulation in people with T1D. Most APs need manual announcement of disturbances such as exercise, preventing full automation and imposing an additional burden on people with T1D. Although exercise is recommended for improving the quality of life and health of people with T1D, the challenge of maintaining euglycemia during and immediately following physical activity prevents many patients from exercising. Physical activity can induce hyper- or hypoglycemia, depending on the type, duration, and intensity of physical activity. The lack of first-principles models of glucose and insulin dynamics during exercise prevents quantification of exercise effects on BGC in people with T1D (Kudva et al. 2014). The use of physiological data collected from biometric sensors can help predict the potential of exercise-induced hyper- or hypoglycemia and provide better BGC regulation with an AP. Biometric sensors provide data that enable an AP to detect the onset, intensity, and duration of physical activity in order to compensate for physiological changes that affect glucose and insulin dynamics (Dasanayake et al. 2015). Sensor data can be used to modify the parameters of physiological models by signaling the changing state of the user's metabolism. These data can also be used to detect and discriminate various types of psychological stress (Sevil et al. 2017).

Biometric sensors fall into two main categories: *consumer devices* that are used by the general population for fitness and lifestyle tracking and *medical-grade devices* used by the medical and research communities for patient monitoring. Fitness trackers are usually wristbands or chest bands that report heart rate and other activity indicators including steps taken and calories burned during workout. Heart rate can usually be monitored in real time with measurements taken every second, but more detailed exercise summaries can be viewed via a mobile app or computer software when data are uploaded via Bluetooth or USB connection. Since an AP needs to be informed of the physiological status of the user in real time, the only useful data from fitness trackers would be information that can be streamed in real time. Such data can inform the AP algorithm during exercise and may help mitigate exercise-induced hypoglycemia. Table 2.2 lists some fitness trackers. The Zephyr BioHarness 3 chest band and BioMedia SenseWear armband (Andre et al. 2006) data were used to determine what physiological variables might be useful to include in a future AP system (Turksoy et al. 2017d). A Polar heart rate monitor was used in a study examining the effects of augmenting an AP system with heart rate data (Dasanayake et al. 2015).

Table 2.2 Sensors for physiological (Biometric) variables

ActiGraph wGT3X-BT activity monitor: (ActiGraph) It can be worn on the wrist and also on the waist, ankle, or thigh. It measures acceleration. Its sampling rate is configurable between 30 and 100 Hz, and it has 2GB (120 days) of memory, but it does not have real-time monitoring capability. It is powered by a rechargeable battery that lasts 25 days maximum (at 30 Hz and with wireless disabled). It has Bluetooth and USB connectivity. The device has FDA approval and costs $225. The data analysis software costs $1695
Polar H10 heart rate monitor: (Polar) It is worn on the chest and measures heart rate. Its sampling rate is 1 Hz, it can store data from one training session, and it has real-time monitoring capability via mobile apps. It is powered by a disposable battery that lasts about 400 h. It has Bluetooth connectivity and is compatible with iOS and Android mobile devices. It has FDA approval. It costs $90
Zephyr BioHarness 3 activity + heart rate monitor: (Medtronic–Zephyr was acquired by Covidien that was acquired by Medtronic) A chest band that measures ECG and heart rate at 250 Hz, acceleration at 100 Hz, and respiratory rate at 25 Hz. It can store 500+ hours of data and has real-time monitoring capability via proprietary software. It is powered by a rechargeable battery that lasts between 12 and 24 h while wirelessly transmitting data. It has Bluetooth and USB connectivity as well as Zephyrs proprietary ECHO connectivity. The device has FDA approval and an assessment kit including the biomodule, torso strap, device charger, ECHO gateway, and cables. The BioHarness costs $550, and OmniSense software costs $4000
Empatica E4 wristband: (Empatica) A wristband that measures blood volume pulse (BVP, used to derive heart rate) at 64 Hz, galvanic skin response and skin temperature at 4 Hz, and acceleration at 32 Hz. It can store 60+ hours of data and has real-time monitoring capability via customizable mobile and desktop applications. It is powered by a rechargeable battery that lasts 20+ hours in streaming mode and 36+ hours in memory mode. It has Bluetooth and USB connectivity, and its apps are compatible with both Mac and PC operating systems as well as iOS and Android mobile devices. Data can also be stored, viewed, and shared through a secure cloud platform. The system has FDA approval and costs $1690
Mio Alpha 2 heart rate monitor: (Mio Global) A wristband that measures heart rate at 1 Hz. It can store up to 25 h of data and allows for real-time monitoring capability via mobile apps. It is powered by a rechargeable battery that lasts 20–24 h in workout mode. It has Bluetooth connectivity and is compatible with iOS and Android mobile devices. The device has FDA approval and costs $119
EQ02 LifeMonitor activity + heart rate monitor: (Equivital) A chest band that measures ECG and heart rate at 256 Hz, acceleration between 25 and 250 Hz, respiratory rate, and skin temperature. Galvanic skin response (GSR) and core temperature can be recorded with auxiliary sensors. It has 8GB (lasting about 7 weeks) of memory and allows for real-time monitoring via proprietary mobile and desktop applications. It is powered by a rechargeable battery that lasts 24–48 h depending on its configuration. It has Bluetooth and USB connectivity and is compatible with Android mobile devices and PC operating systems. The device has FDA approval and costs $2500 including real-time monitoring capability, and the data analysis software costs $2200 for start-up and a 1-year subscription
Fitbit Alta HR heart rate monitor: (Fitbit) A wristband that measures heart rate at 1 Hz. It can store 7 days of data, and it allows for real-time monitoring, but it requires manual syncing to its desktop or mobile app to view data history/trends. It is powered by a rechargeable battery that lasts up to 7 days. It has Bluetooth connectivity and is compatible with iOS, Android, and Windows mobile devices. The device has FDA approval and costs $150

(continued)

Table 2.2 (continued)

Garmin vivosmart HR heart rate monitor: (Garmin) A wristband that measures heart rate every 5–10 min during periods of low activity and every few seconds during periods of high activity. It can store 14 days of data, and it allows for real-time monitoring. Although data are synced with the mobile app automatically throughout the day, it is not done continuously, and data history/trends cannot be monitored in real time. It is powered by a rechargeable battery that lasts up to 5 days. It has Bluetooth and ANT+ connectivity and is compatible with iOS, Android, and Windows mobile devices. The device has FDA approval and costs $150
BioStampRC system: (MC10) The BioStamp sensors can be worn on many different parts of the body, including the hand, foot, arm, leg, chest, and lower back. The sensors collect accelerometer and gyroscope data at a frequency of up to 250 Hz and biopotential data at a frequency of up to 1000 Hz. Each sensor has 32 MB of memory and allows for real-time monitoring via a proprietary tablet application. Each sensor is powered by a rechargeable battery that can last for up to 36 h depending on the configuration, but is recommended for 24 h of use. The sensors have Bluetooth connectivity and are compatible with Android mobile devices. Data can also be stored, viewed, and shared through a secure cloud platform. The system has FDA approval and costs $2500 for the evaluation kit, which includes 3 sensors, stickers and contact gel for the sensors, 1 charger, 1 tablet with the pre-installed mobile application, and 3 years of data access
Cricket wearable sensor: (Somaxis) It can be worn on any location on the body. It collects accelerometer/gyroscope data at a frequency of 30 Hz and EXG data at 1000 Hz when streaming data in real time to proprietary Chirp software. The device has 12.5MB of memory and allows for real-time monitoring of EMG and EKG data, while EEG and accelerometer/gyroscope data can only be stored and viewed later. The device is powered by a rechargeable battery that can last for up to 11 h while live-streaming data. It has Bluetooth connectivity and is compatible with iPad. Data can also be stored, viewed, and shared through a secure cloud platform. The device has FDA approval and costs $262.50 for 1 Cricket sensor and 50 disposable electrode patches
Hexoskin Smart Shirt: (Carré Technologies, Inc) The device is worn as a sleeveless or long-sleeved shirt. It collects acceleration data at a frequency of 64 Hz, ECG data at 256 Hz, heart rate and breathing rate at 1 Hz, and it also provides an estimate of energy expenditure in kcal, among other measurements. The shirt can record for more than 600 h and allows for real-time monitoring via mobile apps. It is powered by a rechargeable battery that lasts at least 14 h. The shirt has Bluetooth connectivity and is compatible with iOS and Android. Raw data can be analyzed using several different types of compatible data analysis software, although VivoSense is recommended. The system has FDA approval and costs $399, which includes the shirt with integrated sensors, a Bluetooth recording device, mobile application downloads, and a USB cable for charging and data upload

Wristbands such as Fitbit and Garmin were used in various studies for retrospective analysis of exercise effects.

Biometric sensors used by the medical and research communities provide more variables to describe the physiological state of users during exercise, including heart rate, respiratory rate, tri-axis acceleration, skin temperature, galvanic skin response, heart rate variability (based on ECG data), posture, and blood volume pulse. These devices are usually worn as wristbands or chest bands, and many of them allow for real-time data monitoring through proprietary software. These devices also have higher data fidelity, with measurement frequencies between 30 and 250 times per second. The sensors that allow for real-time monitoring could be incorporated into AP systems in order to provide data that could help predict the onset and type of exercise as well as determine appropriate changes to physiological parameters such as insulin sensitivity. Such information can be used by the AP to mitigate hypoglycemia either immediately following or hours after exercise. Sensors that do not allow for real-time monitoring could be used to retrospectively analyze relationships between different physiological variables in order to create a black-box model of glucose and insulin dynamics during exercise that could then be incorporated into an AP. The ActiGraph wGT3X-BT wireless activity monitor and the Zephyr BioHarness 3 were used in studies examining the effects of augmenting AP systems with heart rate and acceleration data (Turksoy et al. 2017d; Dasanayake et al. 2015; Stenerson et al. 2014b).

Several studies have reported the use of physiological data from biometric sensors to improve the performance of APs during exercise-induced challenges. However, measuring just one biometric variable is not sufficient to accurately detect physical activity and improve an AP system. Multiple biometric sensors should be used along with CGM sensors in order to make a comprehensive assessment of the metabolic state and activities of the user and to mitigate issues associated with sensor failure and dropout, as well as limitations inherent in each type of measurement. For example, the accuracy of accelerometers for detecting different types of exercise is dependent on their placement on the body, and heart rate monitors can be unreliable if the wearer is moving (Dasanayake et al. 2015). Biometric variables are also usually highly correlated, so the method of data analysis used in the AP should be carefully considered.

2.3 Insulin Pumps

CSII was first introduced in the 1970 s as an improved flexible insulin delivery method (Cengiz et al. 2011; Weissberg-Benchell et al. 2003; Lenhard and Reeves 2001). The portable electromechanical pump infuses short-acting insulin into subcutaneous tissue at preselected basal rates, with user-determined bolus dosing for meals and hyperglycemic episodes (Pickup and Keen 2002). It allows for variable basal insulin rates to cope with circadian rhythms, exercise, and stress caused by illness or psychological stress, and other factors that affect BGC. Indications for insulin pump therapy include persistently high A1C despite MDI therapy, recurring hypoglycemia and frequent wide glycemic excursions (Schaepelynck et al. 2011). Several types of pumps are available, including the original external pump, which consists of an infusion set connected by tubing to the reservoir device, the sensor-augmented pump (SAP) where CGM communicates directly with the pump, and the implanted pump (Schaepelynck et al. 2011). Not all pumps are approved for use in all countries. The implanted pump is not available in the USA. The implanted pump and catheter are inserted into the abdominal wall and intraperitoneal cavity, respectively, and insulin delivery is determined by a personal pump communicator. These pumps require a highly concentrated insulin with long-term stability at body temperature to accommodate the reservoir in the peritoneal cavity as it cannot be replenished easily (Spaan et al. 2014). Despite limited availability, need for intense patient education, and cost, the benefits of insulin pump therapy outweigh these limitations. The most concerning problem with insulin pumps is the potential for disruption of insulin administration (pump failure, kinked tubing, etc.) with subsequent development of diabetic ketoacidosis due to the short duration of the fast-acting insulin used in pumps (Saboo and Talaviya 2012).

Pump therapy has led to significant reductions in A1C without increasing hypoglycemia (Weissberg-Benchell et al. 2003; Lenhard and Reeves 2001; Pickup and Keen 2002). A retrospective observational analysis comparing CSII and MDI patient groups showed a significant A1C reduction in the CSII cohort, as well as a drop in the number of hypoglycemic excursions (Cohen et al. 2013). However, A1C improvement decreased over time, indicating the need for patient reeducation and re-engagement (Cohen et al. 2013). Some studies have reported a decline in depressive symptoms, anxiety and increased adherence to the insulin regimen while on CSII (Weissberg-Benchell et al. 2003).

Various insulin pumps are available in the market. The MiniMed 530G diabetes management system by Medtronic includes the MiniMed 530G insulin pump fully integrated with Enlite CGM. Animas manufactures two different diabetes management systems: the Vibe system and the OneTouch Ping system. The Animas Vibe system has a Vibe insulin pump fully integrated with Dexcom G4 CGM. This system is indicated for use in patients as young as 2 years old. The Animas OneTouch Ping system includes the OneTouch Ping insulin pump along with the OneTouch Ping meter remote which acts as both a glucose meter and a wireless remote to control the pump from up to 10 feet away. Recently the manufacturer of Animas pumps announced that the manufacturing and sale of the Vibe and the OneTouch Ping systems are discontinued and the company is exiting the insulin pump business. The Omnipod insulin management system manufactured by Insulet consists of the pod and the personal diabetes manager (PDM). The pod is a small patch with a built-in insulin reservoir that delivers insulin continuously as it communicates wirelessly with the PDM in a 5-foot range. Tandem manufactures three different insulin pumps: the t:slim X2, the t:slim G4, and the t:flex. These pumps are all powered by rechargeable batteries. The t:slim X2 is the smallest available insulin pump with a 300-unit insulin capacity and a touch screen interface. The t:slim G4 is the smallest available CGM-enabled insulin pump, and it is fully integrated with Dexcom G4 CGM. The t:flex is also smaller than other pumps on the market, and it has the largest insulin reservoir (480 units). Table 2.3 provides additional information about these devices.

Several companies have integrated a CGM and an insulin pump to build SAP therapy systems. Studies evaluating SAP have shown that patients utilizing these systems have improved A1C. SAP therapy in adults and children with T1D was associated with a greater A1C reduction compared to injection therapy (Bergenstal et al. 2010). Moreover, sensor use of $\geq$80% time was associated with an almost doubled reduction in A1C when compared to the A1C reduction when the CGM sensor was used 41–80% of the time (Bergenstal et al. 2010). A study comparing outcomes of patients using a conventional pump with SMBG to those using SAP therapy reported a significant difference in A1C reduction in the SAP cohort (Schae-

Table 2.3 Insulin pumps

MiniMed 530G with Enlite sensor: (Medtronic) The pump is powered by one 1.5 V AAA alkaline battery and has a reservoir capacity of either 180 or 300 units. The basal and bolus delivery accuracy is 5%, and insulin is delivered in increments as small as 0.025 units. The retail price for the pump is $7899. The pump receives glucose data from the sensor via radio signal, and it has USB connectivity for data upload to CareLink software. It has FDA approval for use by patients 16 years and older who are not critically ill, pregnant, or on dialysis. The system provides alerts for low reservoir, missed bolus, and low battery
Animas Vibe with DG4P sensor: (Animas) The pump is powered by one 1.5 V AA lithium battery that lasts 3–4 weeks and has a reservoir capacity of 200 units. The basal and bolus delivery accuracy is 5%, and insulin is delivered in increments as small as 0.025 units for the basal rate and 0.050 units for boluses. The retail price for the pump is $7150. The pump receives glucose data from the DG4P sensor via RF communication, and it has USB connectivity for data upload to diabetes management software. It has FDA approval for use by patients 2 years and older. The system provides audible and vibratory alerts for high and low BG excursions
Animas OneTouch Ping with meter remote: (Animas) The pump is powered by one 1.5 V AA lithium battery that lasts 5–7 weeks and has a reservoir capacity of 200 units. The basal and bolus delivery accuracy is 5%, and insulin is delivered in increments as small as 0.025 units for the basal rate and 0.050 units for boluses. The retail price for the pump is $6662. The pump and meter remote are connected via RF communication, and the pump has USB connectivity for data upload to diabetes management software. The system has FDA approval, and it provides audible and vibratory alerts for high and low BG excursions
Insulet OmniPod: (Insulet) The remote personal diabetes manager (PDM) is powered by 2 AAA alkaline batteries that last about 3 weeks, and the pod has a reservoir capacity of 200 units. The basal and bolus delivery accuracy is 5%, and insulin is delivered in increments as small as 0.050 units. The retail price for a pack of 10 pods is $450 and for the PDM is $1750. The pod and PDM are connected via RF communication. The system has FDA approval. The pod provides audible alerts, and the PDM provides audible and vibratory alerts
Tandem t:slim X2: (Tandem) The pump is powered by a rechargeable battery that lasts up to 7 days and has a reservoir capacity of 300 units. The basal and bolus delivery accuracy is 5%, and insulin is delivered in increments as small as 0.001 units. The retail price for the pump is $4995. It has USB connectivity for data upload to a Mac and PC-compatible app, and it has Bluetooth capability for remote software updates. The system has FDA approval for use by patients 6 years and older using NovoLog or Humalog U-100 insulin. The pod provides visual, audible, and vibratory alerts for low reservoir, low power, incomplete programming action, and for attempts to program outside the maximum and minimum basal and bolus limits
Tandem t:slim G4: (Tandem) The pump is powered by a rechargeable battery that lasts up to 7 days (5 days if used with compatible DG4P sensor) and has a reservoir capacity of 300 units. The basal and bolus delivery accuracy is 5%, and insulin is delivered in increments as small as 0.001 units. The retail price for the pump is $4695. It has USB connectivity for data upload to a Mac and PC-compatible application. The system has FDA approval to be used by patients 12 years and older using NovoLog or Humalog U-100 insulin. The pod provides visual, audible, and vibratory alerts for low reservoir, low power, incomplete programming action, and for attempts to program outside the maximum and minimum basal and bolus limits
Tandem t:flex: (Tandem) The pump is powered by a rechargeable battery that lasts up to 4 days and has a reservoir capacity of 480 units. The basal and bolus delivery accuracy is 5%, and insulin is delivered in increments as small as 0.001 units. The retail price for the pump is $4500. It has USB connectivity for data upload to a Mac and PC-compatible application. The system has FDA approval for use by patients 12 years and older using NovoLog or Humalog U-100 insulin. The pod provides visual, audible, and vibratory alerts for low reservoir, low power, incomplete programming action, and for attempts to program outside the maximum and minimum basal and bolus limits

pelynck et al. 2011). Most studies have also shown that SAP therapy is not associated with increased frequency of nor elimination of hypoglycemia (Schaepelynck et al. 2011).

Most pumps are capable of receiving external signals to adjust insulin flow rates by using proprietary communication protocols. Hence, they can be used in AP systems with secure communications.

2.4 Controllers

The control algorithm of the AP is responsible for calculating the optimal basal and bolus insulin and/or glucagon dose or carbohydrate to be ingested, based on the patients glucose concentration estimates and physiological properties, to reach the target glucose range. Proportional–integral–derivative (PID), model predictive control (MPC), generalized predictive control (GPC, adaptive control), and knowledge-based fuzzy logic control algorithms have been used for BGC regulation (Doyle et al. 2014; Turksoy et al. 2017a).

The difference between the desired glucose concentration (the set point or reference BGC value or the desired glucose range for euglycemia) and the CGM readings generates an error signal, which is the main input to all controllers. The classical PID control tries to minimize the difference between the reference and measured CGM by adjusting insulin infusion rates without any physiological information about glucose/insulin dynamics. Controller parameters can be tuned to change the aggressiveness of the controller in response to glucose variations. Proportional (P) action in PID provides instantaneous response, integral (I) action eliminates final steady-state offset between desired and measured values of the controlled variable, and derivative (D) action enables anticipatory response based on the slope of the current change. It cannot accommodate constraints on insulin infusion rates and changes in infusion rates in consecutive adjustments. It is based on the error between the current CGM value and the reference BGC value and cannot use predictions of future BGC trajectories based on past insulin infusions and future hypothetical infusions to find the current optimal insulin infusion rate. One appeal of PID control was the similarity of insulin release profile from the pancreas in response to a sharp increase in BGC to the response of a proportional–derivative controller to a step change in an input. While PID control has been used in various industries for over 80 years, the traditional PID is no match for the dynamics of the human body, a nonlinear system with time-varying parameters. Several estimators and extensions provided a comprehensive PID to address these limitations for its use in APs (Steil and Rebrin 2008; Steil 2013; Kanderian and Steil 2010; Palerm 2011).

MPC and GPC algorithms address both limitations (prediction of future BGC and accommodation of constraints) in a systematic way. They use mathematical models for prediction of future BGCs. With every new measurement, not only the difference between current glucose measurement and the reference value is minimized, but also a sequence of future insulin infusion rates is computed over a control horizon that minimizes the "error" between future glucose concentrations (predicted by the model) and the desired glucose concentrations. Development of an MPC algorithm that uses a physical (compartmental) model requires detailed physiological information about the human body and glucose/insulin dynamics because the whole control algorithm is based on equations derived from first principles. The alternative is to use data-driven empirical dynamic models. The models used can be general models for a population, model with parameters adjusted for each individual, models for individuals that are updated daily based on the model performance on the previous day or recursively updated models at each sampling time when new data are received from sensors. The accuracy of predictions improve as the frequency of updating the model parameters increases. In a GPC algorithm with an empirical input–output subject model, parameters can be updated with every new measurement to track dynamic changes in the human body over time, enabling an adaptive control framework that uses a model that expresses the current state of the patient accurately.

Knowledge-based fuzzy logic controllers mimic and automate the decision-making process of a clinician based on the current state of the subject. Several if-then rules are defined to calculate insulin infusion rates by using this "qualitative" model rather than mathematical models. One of the challenges of such knowledge-based systems is the formulation of an insulin delivery decision for a set of conditions experienced by the subject that have not been considered by the system developers yet. Rule-based systems can be easily updated to accommodate such previously not considered states. A second challenge is conflict resolution when some rules suggest actions that contradict the suggestions made by other rules. The possibility of conflicting decisions increases as the number of rules is increased. The conflicts can be resolved by assigning different priority levels to various rules so that rules with higher priorities can override decisions made based on rules with lower priority.

Chapter 3
Factors Affecting Blood Glucose Concentration and Challenges to AP Systems

Abstract An AP system is challenged by several factors such as meals, exercise, sleep and stress that may have significant effects on glucose dynamics in the body. In this chapter, the relationship between these factors and the glucose dynamics are discussed. Most AP systems are based only on glucose measurements. These systems usually require manual inputs or adjustments by the users about the occurrences of some of these factors such as meals and exercise. Alternatively, multivariable AP systems have been proposed that use biometric variables in addition to glucose measurements to indicate the presence of these factors without a need for manual user input. The effects of different types of insulin as well as use of glucagon in AP systems is also discussed. The chapter includes a discussion of time delays in glucose sensors that affect the performance of predictive hypoglycemia alarm systems and APs.

Keywords Meals · Exercise · Stress · Sleep · Hypoglycemia · Insulin · Glucagon

Glucose is the primary source of energy for the body. Many organs can also use fat and proteins as the source of energy when BGC is too low, except the brain and nervous system that consume exclusively glucose for functioning. Consequently, low BGC affects the operation of the brain and has drastic effects on rational thinking. Hypoglycemia can cause disorientation, fainting, diabetic coma and even death. Hypoglycemia is a major concern and source of fear for people with T1D. While hypoglycemia has important effects in the short term, large excursions in BGC, and long periods of high BGC cause long-term damage to the vascular system, leading to cardiovascular diseases, kidney failure, neuropathy, retinopathy and blindness, skin ulcers, and difficulties in wound healing that may lead to amputations.

Studies have reported that the use of AP would reduce the fear of hypoglycemia since the AP can adjust insulin infusion rates based on glucose levels. Automated shutdown of insulin flow based on hypoglycemia predictions is an effective safety feature. Most hypoglycemia prediction and AP systems rely only on CGM information. Several factors that occur during the daily lives of people with T1D may have

A. Cinar and K. Turksoy, *Advances in Artificial Pancreas Systems*,
SpringerBriefs in Bioengineering, https://doi.org/10.1007/978-3-319-72245-0_3

drastic and rapid effects on BGC. Meals, exercise, sleep, and acute psychological stress (MESS) influence BGC. Meals cause rapid spikes in BGC, aerobic exercise increases the sensitivity to insulin and causes rapid declines in BGC, psychological stress reduces the sensitivity to insulin and causes temporary increases in BGC, and sleep may cause dawn phenomenon and poor sleep affects BGC trends the following day. While the effects of all these factors can be noticed in CGM data, other variables may indicate their presence sooner, provide valuable information to an AP, and enable anticipatory decisions to counter the effects of MESS.

3.1 Meals

Food consumption causes rapid increase in BGC. Several factors influence glycemic response to food, including food form (i.e., solid, liquid), degree of cooking and processing, macronutrient composition, fiber, anti-nutrients (e.g., amylase inhibitors), amount of food consumed at one time, meal frequency, rate of ingestion, and physiologic effects (Wong and Jenkins 2007; Shils et al. 1998). These factors impact the rate of digestion and absorption, and subsequent glycemic response that must be predicted by AP systems.

Absorption of nutrients is related to the inherent qualities of the nutrients, their interactions with each other and with nonabsorbable food components (i.e., fiber) (Shils et al. 1998). To optimize glycemic control, these factors can be modified to reduce the rate of nutrient absorption and flatten the glycemic response. Macronutrient composition and indigestible components of food can influence nutrient absorption. Carbohydrates (CHO) belong to one of three groups: sugars (mono- and disaccharides), starch, and fiber (Franz et al. 2002). The body breaks down all CHO, with the exception of fiber, into monosaccharides for absorption during digestion. The rise in BGC varies based on the type of sugars consumed. The greatest increase in BGC has been observed for glucose and maltose, while fructose produces a smaller increase, and sucrose and lactose cause more moderate increase (Frost et al. 2003; Nuttall et al. 1984; Pettus et al. 2013). Although fiber is resistant to digestion by dietary enzymes, it plays an important role in the rate of nutrient absorption. Soluble fiber, in particular, delays gastric emptying, slows nutrient absorption, and flattens postprandial BGC response (Jenkins et al. 1978; Holt et al. 1979). Digestion and absorption of glucose are also slowed by intake of dietary fat (Collier et al. 1984; Frost et al. 2003). Co-ingestion of CHO and fat flattens postprandial BGC response but does not significantly affect postprandial insulin levels (Collier et al. 1984; Frost et al. 2003). Protein and CHO consumed together reduce the increase in BGC and increase insulin secretion compared to CHO alone; however, protein has not been demonstrated to slow the absorption of CHO (Nuttall et al. 1984).

Because a multitude of factors influence glycemic response, it is not possible to predict the physiologic effect of food based on chemical composition. An index of the physiological effects of food, the glycemic index, supplements data on chemical composition of foods (Shils et al. 1998; Jenkins et al. 1981). Glycemic index can aid in insulin dosing predictions. Many people with T1D estimate the CHO amount in their meals and some make adjustments to account for the effects of fat and protein content for computing the insulin bolus. The same approach can work when meal information is manually entered to the AP. Two alternatives can be used to eliminate manual entry to the AP. The first is to develop elaborate meal assessment techniques such as taking images of food to be consumed and analyzing meal contents from images, and sensing jaw or wrist motions to automate meal predictions. The second alternative is to develop meal detection techniques by using CGM data and algorithms to manage boluses based on the estimated CHO content. AP systems must be flexible to accommodate all combinations of food products ingested. Determining all these information and manually entering them to an AP is challenging. Furthermore, people may even forget to enter the meal information altogether. While early APs have relied on manual meal information, several research groups are considering APs that do not require manual meal entry and mitigating meal effects by using machine learning techniques to detect ingestion of a meal (Cameron et al. 2009; Turksoy et al. 2016; Samadi et al. 2017) and estimate the amount of CHO consumed (Samadi et al. 2017) for computing insulin boluses.

3.2 Exercise and Physical Activities

Physical activities include a brisk walking to catch a bus, housekeeping activities, individual daily exercise routines, and group sports. It could be a planned activity, often referred to as exercise, with known characteristics or a spontaneous event with no a priori knowledge of its structure or intensity. Exercise is quantified by frequency (how often), intensity (how hard), duration (how long), and type (aerobic, anaerobic, or mixed anaerobic and aerobic). Exercise in people with T1D is associated with multiple challenges. In normal physiology, rate of glucose appearance (Ra) and rate of glucose disappearance (Rd) reach equilibrium during exercise, largely influenced by changes in insulin, glucagon, growth hormone, and catecholamines. In people with T1D, the equilibrium between Ra and Rd is impaired by a number of factors, including altered counterregulation and inability to reduce or increase insulin delivery to the portal circulation (Riddell et al. 2015). Mild and moderate-intensity exercise may necessitate a reduction in insulin infusion, while more intense activities may necessitate an increase in insulin infusion, especially during early recovery (Riddell et al. 2015). There is a reduction in insulin secretion at the onset of moderate to vigorous/maximum-intensity exercise in people without T1D and a rise in insulin secretion at the end of vigorous-maximal exercise (Riddell et al. 2015). During high-intensity exercise, more glucose is used because there is a greater muscle recruitment and greater energy expenditure. APs must be able to recognize activities that increase the intensity and compensate accordingly (Peake et al. 2014). The integration of biomarkers, such as serum lactate levels, into AP models may assist in determining exercise intensity and predicting BGC.

Altered physiological responses during exercise can result in hyper- and hypoglycemia. Hypoglycemia remains as the limiting factor in adopting a physically active lifestyle among people with T1D. The primary factors associated with hypoglycemia during exercise include the frequency, intensity, and duration of exercise, circulating insulin levels (insulin on board), and availability of supplemental CHOs. Athletes with T1D often must go through a trial-and-error scenario to tailor their insulin and CHO administration to each workout. Current exercise guidelines suggest that each person develop a personalized plan by using the standards of care (Galassetti and Riddell 2013) as an initiation point. This allows the individual to gain experience with insulin dose adjustments and CHO intake for various types of exercise. This laborious process is made more difficult due to intra-individual variations in glucose responses to exercise such as early versus delayed hypoglycemia. A recent consensus report provides valuable information on exercise management in T1D (Riddell et al. 2017). While an individual with a well-defined exercise routine can mitigate the effects of exercise on BGC variations based on personal knowledge, the automation of these decisions with an AP will necessitate timely and accurate information about the presence and characteristics of a physical activity (Riddell et al. 2015). An AP should have the ability to anticipate BGC levels and adjust insulin and/or glucagon dosing or suggest rescue CHO ingestion to rapid changes in BGC based on the characteristics of the physical activity performed. This necessitates a multivariable approach that can inform the AP about the exercise well before changes in BGC and algorithms that can detect and discriminate the physical activity accurately (Turksoy et al. 2015, 2017d).

Research on the use of AP during exercise are limited, and some studies have included periods of structured exercise as part of their AP experiment protocols (Hovorka et al. 2010; Murphy et al. 2011; Russell et al. 2012; Breton et al. 2012, 2014; El-Khatib et al. 2014; Elleri et al. 2014; Turksoy et al. 2013b, 2014a; Van Bon et al. 2012; Garg et al. 2012; Sherr et al. 2013; Breton et al. 2017). Several challenges must be addressed for developing APs that can regulate BGC variations during and after a variety of physical activities. Measured variables that provide information to detect and classify the type and intensity of physical activities must be determined. This information is useful in adjusting the models used by the AP for BGC estimations. Sensor type and placement location are also important. It is critical to detect and discriminate concurrent MESS activities such as exercise and psychological stress since they have different effects on BGC changes. Since the number of wearable devices used should be kept to a minimum, the determination of variables that can provide reliable information about the exercise being performed and the presence of other MESS factors is necessary. The AP must have models that can predict the effects of various types, intensities and durations of physical activity, including intense activity bouts in which the variables are constantly changing, such as starting and stopping in group sports, or long distance running or biking. Multivariable APs with modules for physical activity detection and diagnosis will have a better chance to maintain BGC in the target range during and after exercise.

3.3 Psychological Stress

Psychological stress can be grouped as *chronic* stress and *acute stress*. Since the effects of chronic stress such as depression may not change for long periods of time, the AP can handle its effects on BGC variations. Acute psychological stress is caused by sudden unexpected events such as learning bad news (loss of job) or sudden catastrophic event (fire in the kitchen and traffic accident). This results in sudden changes in insulin sensitivity and causes challenges to the AP, especially when the AP relies only on CGM operation. The focus of the discussion will be on acute psychological stress for AP design. Also, it is common to refer to physical activity as *physiological* stress. In this book, we will use the term stress to refer to acute psychological stress.

The relationship between stress and BGC dynamics is complicated. Stress can affect BGC in people with T1D (Marcovecchio and Chiarelli 2012; Gonder-Frederick et al. 1990; Hanson and Pichert 1986; Halford et al. 1990; Chida and Hamer 2008; Hilliard et al. 2016; Baucom et al. 2015; Frenzel et al. 1988; Surwit and Schneider 1993; Moberg et al. 1994). It can increase BGC levels (Ghosal et al. 2015) due to the release of catecholamines and glucocorticoids, inducing insulin resistance. Thus, more insulin is required to lower BGC into the target range (Ward et al. 2011) during stressful situations. Activation of hormones by psychological stress or anaerobic exercise can increase glucose production and reduce sensitivity to insulin, while medium-intensity aerobic exercise increases sensitivity to insulin and causes hypoglycemia (Riddell et al. 2015; Colberg and Edelman 2008). The magnitude and duration of stress effects on BGC varies for different individuals (Riazi et al. 2004) and is affected by age (Hilliard et al. 2016), sex (Kelly et al. 2008; Kajantie and Phillips 2006) and the presence of concurrent MESS events (Wiesli et al. 2005).

The concurrent high-intensity physical activity and psychological stress such as racing (as opposed to training—physical activity without psychological stress) necessitates the detection of both physical activity and stress, since they affect insulin sensitivity in opposite directions (Perkins and Riddell 2006). Athletes report that while they have hypoglycemia after training, they have hyperglycemia after a competition when they perform a similar physical activity (Colberg and Edelman 2008). This is especially problematic when the pre-competition BGC is elevated; the athlete may administer some insulin to lower BGC, while still allowing a buffer for a possible exercise-induced hypoglycemia. While the effects of chronic stress have been studied in people with T1D, the impact of acute psychological stress in management of glucose levels with AP systems in people with T1D is an open research problem (Gonder-Frederick et al. 2016). An AP must be able to assess changes in stress in combination with exercise to maintain target BCG levels.

3.4 Sleep

Individuals with T1D have altered sleep architecture with less time spent in deep sleep and more time in shallow sleep, and the reduction in deep sleep is associated with poorer glycemic control (Perfect et al. 2012; Feupe et al. 2013; Jauch-Chara et al. 2008). Changes in sleep patterns are common in adolescents with T1D and sleep disturbances have been associated with poorer glycemic control management in this population (Yeshayahu and Mahmud 2010; Estrada et al. 2012; Koren et al. 2015; Jaser and Ellis 2016; McDonough et al. 2017; Turner et al. 2016). T1D is often characterized by unpredictable periods of hypoglycemia and hypoglycemic unawareness especially during sleep, leading to fear of hypoglycemia and risk of complications. The fear of hypoglycemia during sleep and its serious medical complications adversely affects sleep patterns of people with T1D and their family members (Barnard et al. 2016). Most sleep studies have been conducted in sleep laboratories, an environment that can affect the natural sleep patterns of subjects. Few studies that captured data on nocturnal continuous glucose concentrations and sleep stage in people with T1D in real-world conditions have also confirmed the trends in BGC variations (Feupe et al. 2013).

Dawn phenomenon refers to a rise in BGC during the early morning hours of sleep. This BGC rise can cause poor glycemic control after waking up and during the day for people with T1D (Forlenza et al. 2017). Pronounced BGC increases caused by dawn phenomenon may cause challenges to the AP.

Readings of glucose sensors used in CGMs can be affected when pressure is exerted in the region where the sensor is inserted to subcutaneous tissue. CGMs rely on adequate blood flow to the interstitial space for accurate measurement. Pressure applied to tissue in the immediate vicinity of a sensor may decrease blood flow and oxygen tension (Mensh et al. 2013). This pressure-induced sensor attenuation (PISA) can occur during sleep when the person rotates her/his body and exerts pressure on the sensor location (Baysal et al. 2014). Since the variation in CGM readings is not caused by a metabolic change, any adjustments in insulin infusion rates could cause real variations in BCG. Sensor readings would return to their correct values when the pressure is lifted as the person changes the body position. Detection of PISA and mitigation of its potential effects must be achieved by an AP. Another potential reason of CGM inaccuracies during sleep is temperature-induced physiological fluctuations. Temperature affects both subcutaneous oxygen tension and sensor output current (Mensh et al. 2013). Lying on CGM sensors as well as being under a blanket will likely warm the area around the CGMs and will cause increased sensors readings. Use of skin or near-body temperature measurements in an AP can decrease the risk associated with temperature fluctuations around the CGMs (Turksoy et al. 2017d).

3.5 Hypoglycemia

The risk of hypoglycemia is a real concern for people with T1D (Halimi 2010). Hypoglycemia poses a challenge and an opportunity to enhance the value of the AP since it is expected that the AP must adjust insulin infusion rates to prevent hypoglycemia. The fear of hypoglycemia due to unexpected events and the inability to recognize the occurrence of hypoglycemia either because of compromised rational thinking or not waking up to hypoglycemia alarms while sleeping results in many people preferring to maintain the BGC at higher levels than necessary. In a recent survey, 33% of adults with T1D and T2D (n = 1,848) were very worried about hypoglycemia and thus maintained their BGC in the hyperglycemic range. The average number of emergency visits and hospitalizations per patient per month was 0.65 and 0.47, respectively, and 10% of the patients reported work absence during the previous 12 months because of hypoglycemia (Willis et al. 2013). In addition, 80% of the participants stated that they would value a device that would warn them about an upcoming hypoglycemia episode. The fear of low BGC in T1D may induce overeating and lead to hyperglycemia. Alleviating the hypoglycemia fear with APs would lower the number of complications and health care costs caused by extended periods of hyperglycemia. APs include a hypoglycemia alarm system that could warn individuals that are trending toward hypoglycemia and prevent hypogylcemia by adjusting insulin infusion, and by using glucagon or recommending CHO consumption to raise the BGC if suspension of insulin infusion is insufficient to prevent pending hypoglycemia, then resume insulin infusion when the BGC returns to target range.

3.6 Insulin

The pancreas regulates BGC by secreting hormones into the bloodstream in response to changes in the body. When the BGC of a healthy person rises after a meal, the beta cells in the islets of Langerhans located in the pancreas are stimulated to release insulin that is collected by the surrounding capillaries and introduced to the bloodstream. Insulin lowers BGC by suppressing endogenous glucose production in the liver, promoting glucose disposal via glycogen production in the liver, and distributing glucose to cells in the body.

Rapid-acting insulin analogs (RAIs) transformed diabetes treatment due to their favorable insulin action profile as compared to regular human insulin (Mudaliar et al. 1999; Howey et al. 1994). The RAIs allowed patients to inject or infuse insulin with meals rather than injecting a half hour prior to meals. While RAI action profiles are better than regular insulin they are not fast enough to adequately mimic the physiological post-meal insulin secretion pattern in healthy subjects. Lispro, Novolog, or Apidra are the current types of insulin used. As experience with RAI use increased, their limitations were noticed. Despite the faster onset of action and shorter duration of action as compared to regular insulin, insulin action studies indicate that the onset of action of RAIs is still too slow, with a peak action approximately 90–130 min after subcutaneous injection, leading to exaggerated postprandial BGC excursions and tendency to late postprandial hypoglycemia due to their prolonged action (Swan et al. 2008, 2009). The negative effect of the slow and relatively long action of RAIs has become even more problematic for the AP, inherent from a system that delivers insulin after the BGC starts to rise and stretches the insulin delivery over the course of a few hours rather than manually infusing a pre-meal bolus over a few minutes (Weinzimer et al. 2008; Steil et al. 2006). The slow insulin action of RAI became an important obstacle for achieving optimal performance of fully automated APs. This gave significant momentum to research in ultra-fast acting insulins that can keep up with the pace of the AP and improve control of BGC particularly after meals.

Ultra-fast acting insulin studies focused on changing the molecular structure of insulin to accelerate its action or adjunct methods to deliver insulin faster into the circulation (Cengiz 2013; Heinemann and Muchmore 2012). A novel insulin infusion site warming device, the InsuPatch, has been shown to accelerate insulin absorption and action by increasing blood flow to the infusion area and is now being tested in the closed-loop systems (Cengiz et al. 2013, 2014). Similar results are reported when RAIs are injected or infused in a pre-treated site with recombinant human hyaluronidase, hylenex, that has been shown to increase the permeability of the extracellular matrix in the subcutaneous area (Vaughn and Muchmore 2011). The follow up hylenex studies are designed for testing the insulin action when the RAI is co-formulated with hylenex to improve diffusion and dispersion of insulin, eliminating the need for hylenex pre-injection into the infusion site (Morrow et al. 2013). The randomized, crossover clinical study to investigate the favorable insulin action accelerator effect of hylenex pre-treatment and insulin–hylenex co-formulation on the AP is ongoing.

The Diaport intraperitoneal infusion set is an alternative to deliver insulin faster into the circulation. This system includes a port that is implanted in the abdominal wall, to which an intraperitoneal catheter is connected on one side and an external insulin pump on the other side. The insulin from the pump is infused to the peritoneal vascular plexus directly bypassing the subcutaneous tissue (Liebl et al. 2009). While the data for the Diaport system efficacy have not been widely published, it is already incorporated into the AP in the research setting in Europe.

Peripheral delivery of insulin is not physiologic, but is the best current option. The predominant problem related to this insulin delivery system is delay in action due to subcutaneous absorption and lack of liver metabolism, thus the potential for hyper- or hypoglycemia (Pettus et al. 2013). Other hormones are important in maintaining glucose levels, such as glucagon, and glucagon-like peptide-1 (GLP-1), but glucagon and insulin are the only hormones currently under investigation for use in APs (Bakhtiani et al. 2013).

3.7 Glucagon

When the BGC of a healthy person drops below a certain value, insulin secretion is curtailed and the alpha cells in the islets of Langerhans are stimulated to release glucagon that is collected by the surrounding capillaries. Glucagon is a counterregulatory hormone that stimulates hepatic glucose production by activating glycogenolysis followed by gluconeogenesis, while suppressing glycogenesis and glycolysis (Taleb et al. 2017). While insulin acts to prevent ketoacidosis and hyperglycemia, glucagon acts to prevent hypoglycemia. Ketoacidosis and hypoglycemia have the potential to be fatal if not treated promptly, whereas hyperglycemia causes long-term cardiovascular complications.

Glucagon also affects the cardiovascular, renal, pulmonary, and gastrointestinal systems. Glucagon secretion is regulated by glucose and nutrient sensing by alpha cells, autocrine and paracrine factors in the islets of Langerhans, and through the autonomic nervous system (Taleb et al. 2017). Glucagon is known to be poorly regulated in diabetes. People with uncontrolled T1D have been found to have increased basal, fasting, and postprandial glucagon levels (Taleb et al. 2017). Glucagon response to hypoglycemia in T1D also decreases gradually over time and with recurrent hypoglycemic events. In normal physiology, glucagon, and insulin secretion are closely coordinated and changes in both hormones in the portal system direct the hepatic control of glucose metabolism. In T1D, glucose metabolism fails due to hepatic resistance to insulin and glucagon, insufficient amounts of insulin, and beta cell failure (Taleb et al. 2017).

AP systems that regulate BGC by using only insulin can be limited in their ability to react to low BGC. Hence, dual-hormone AP systems that use both insulin and glucagon are appealing. Two challenges in the use of glucagon are the added complexity of the AP system (two reservoirs and pumps, more complex control algorithm, challenges in delivery) and the lack of a long-term stable glucagon that can be used in AP systems under free-living conditions. Research is progressing in both fronts to enable the development of dual-hormone AP systems.

3.8 Glucose Sensor Signal Accuracy and Delay

In general, the accuracy of CGM sensors is becoming adequate for use in the AP. The major problems include the lag between interstitial and blood glucose, need for more frequent BGC information, missing signals or outliers due to device failure or dislodging, and variability between subjects. Most problems occur because glucose samples are from the interstitium rather than capillary blood. During rapidly changing conditions such as exercise, interstitial glucose, and BGC can be markedly different (Rebrin et al. 1999). Due to the blood-to-interstitial glucose transport, coupled with sensor processing time, there is an inherent time lag. CGM readings lag BGC readings by 4–10 min (Wentholt et al. 2007). Lastly, CGMs experience transient loss of sensitivity due to deterioration of the sensor and random noise (Diabetes Research in Children Network 2008).

Chapter 4
Modeling Glucose and Insulin Concentration Dynamics

Abstract Modeling of glucose and insulin concentration dynamics are discussed, and two different modeling approaches are presented. Physiological models describe the glucose and insulin dynamics with differential equations and physiological rules based on detailed understanding of the glucose and insulin dynamics, mass transfer and reaction kinetics. The chapter outlines progress in physiological modeling over the years. Alternatively, data-driven empirical modeling techniques have also been used to relate the effects of various measured inputs on glucose and insulin dynamics. The advantage of the latter is ease of model development with less information about glucose and insulin dynamics, and rapid model development and updating. Several empirical model types are presented and the technical steps to develop and evaluate them are outlined.

Keywords Modeling · Glucose/Insulin dynamics · Physiological models
Empirical models · Time series models · State space models
Multivariable models

The dynamics of glucose and insulin concentrations can be expressed by using various modeling paradigms, as appropriate for the intended use of the model. Compartmental models based on first principles are used for simulating BGC and insulin dynamics accurately. Input–output models as state-space, transfer function, or time series models are more useful in designing AP control algorithms, hypogylcemia prediction systems, and AP fault detection and diagnosis algorithms.

4.1 Physiological Models

Physiological models use the regulatory mechanisms of glucose and other metabolites to develop mathematical relations expressed by algebraic and ordinary differ-

A. Cinar and K. Turksoy, *Advances in Artificial Pancreas Systems*,
SpringerBriefs in Bioengineering, https://doi.org/10.1007/978-3-319-72245-0_4

ential equations. They are usually compartmental models, generated by dividing the body into several compartments to represent the distribution of glucose and/or insulin in organs or tissues (Carson and Cobelli 2014). A compartment (organ) itself can be divided into multiple regions if mass transfer limitations occur within the compartment. Mass balance equations are written around each compartment, resulting in a set of differential equations that are solved simultaneously. These models also include pharmacokinetic diagrams of exogenously administered insulin and glucose absorption from the gastrointestinal track following a meal consumption. Since blood glucose regulation is a highly nonlinear and complex process, some physiological models are representative of an "average" person under specific and disturbance-free conditions (Sorensen 1985; Puckett 1992; Agar et al. 2006). Most physiological models are too complex for use in control systems but they are valuable in simulators. Recent work in simulator development accommodated many nonlinearities and developed a number of "virtual patients" by identifying the model parameters based on data from a small number of subjects, generating distribution functions for model parameters from these data, and using these distributions for computing the model parameters for virtual patients (Dalla Man et al. 2014).

A frequently used physiological model in the literature to describe the glucose–insulin interactions in the human body (Bergman 1989) is the so-called minimal model (MM) (Bergman et al. 1979, 1989). The model was originally proposed to interpret plasma glucose and insulin concentrations following an intravenous glucose tolerance test (IVGTT) in healthy subjects. In IVGTT test, subjects are injected with an intravenously administered glucose load, and the plasma glucose and insulin concentrations are measured frequently until the effect of the glucose load subsides. In the MM model, glucose–insulin interactions in the body are described with a two-compartment model that is represented by three ordinary differential equations and a few parameters (Fig. 4.1). Plasma glucose dynamics, plasma insulin dynamics, and insulin concentration in a remote inaccessible compartment are included in the

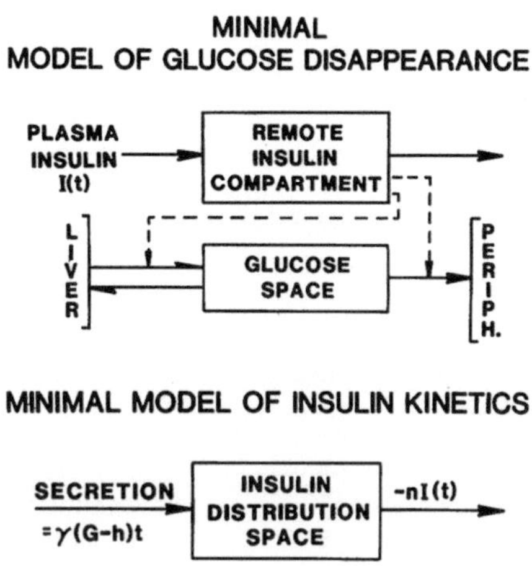

Fig. 4.1 Bergman's minimal Glucose/Insulin model

model. A subject's insulin sensitivity (quantitative expression of the response of the body to insulin) and glucose effectiveness (ability of glucose to stimulate its own uptake and suppress its own release) are established by the MM. The accuracy of the MM has been debated by many researchers (Weber et al. 1989; Quon et al. 1994; Caumo et al. 1999; De Gaetano and Arino 2000). For instance, in Quon et al. (1994), overestimation of the effect of glucose on glucose uptake and underestimation of the contribution of incremental insulin by the MM are reported. Also, stability problems of the MM have been revealed (De Gaetano and Arino 2000). The MM does not admit equilibrium, and the insulin concentration in the remote compartment increases without bounds for some situations (De Gaetano and Arino 2000). The MM and its extensions remain as the most popular physiological model, because of its simple structure and minimum number of parameters that are easily identifiable.

The original MM model (Bergman et al. 1979) has been extended to include three subsystems (glucose, insulin, and glucagon) (Cobelli et al. 1982; Cobelli and Mari 1983). The effect of glucagon on glucose metabolism is included explicitly in this extended model. In the extended MM model, the glucose and glucagon subsystems are each depicted with a single compartment, while the insulin subsystem consists of five compartments (plasma, liver, interstitial insulin, stored, and promptly releasable pancreatic insulin). The glucose subsystem considers glucose production and uptake by liver, renal excretion, insulin-dependent and insulin-independent glucose utilization.

In a recent study, the MM has been modified to provide the metabolic portrait of a whole population (Vicini and Cobelli 2001). Originally, the MM was proposed to describe the glucose metabolism of a single person. In Vicini and Cobelli (2001), the authors proposed a Bayesian approach for the population-based minimal model. Distributions of population insulin sensitivity and glucose effectiveness are computed using IVGTT data from 16 healthy people. Then, the mean and standard deviations of these population distributions are used as prior information for individual analysis.

The original MM does not consider the absorption of exogenously administered insulin and the CHO absorption from the gut after a food consumption. An improvement of MM is proposed by adding intestinal glucose absorption to the model (Lehmann and Deutsch 1992). This model attempts to reflect the underlying pathophysiology of insulin action and CHO absorption in quantitative terms such as insulin sensitivity, volume of glucose and insulin distribution, and maximal rate of gastric emptying in people with T1D. Similar to the original MM, a single glucose compartment is utilized. However, glucose enters into the compartment by intestinal absorption and hepatic production, and is removed by insulin-independent glucose utilization in the red blood cells, insulin-dependent utilization in the liver and periphery, and renal glucose excretion.

Hovorka et al. (2002, 2004) have extended the MM by including an additional subsystem for insulin action (Fig. 4.2). This subsystem considers the effect of insulin on glucose distribution/transport, glucose disposal, and endogenous glucose production. The glucose subsystem includes renal glucose excretion, endogenous glucose production, insulin-independent glucose flux, and intestinal absorption. The insulin subsystem describes the subcutaneous insulin absorption and is partitioned into two

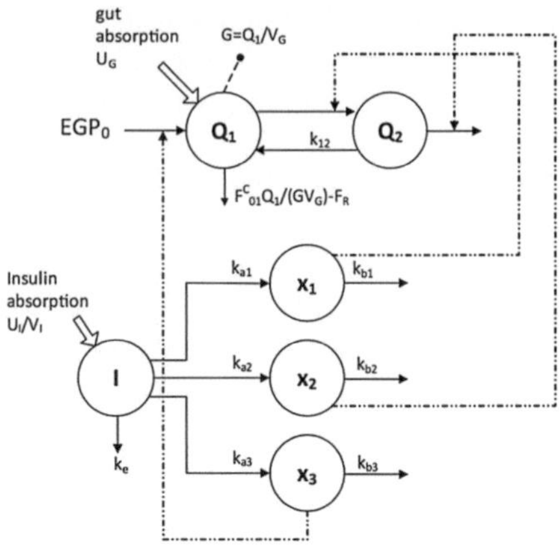

Fig. 4.2 Hovorka's Glucose/Insulin model (Hovorka et al. 2004) ©2004 Institute of Physics and Engineering in Medicine. Reproduced by permission of IOP Publishing.

compartments. The model parameters are identified by using a dual-tracer dilution method during an IVGTT.

A more extensive physiological model was developed by Sorensen (1985). The body was divided into seven compartments representing various body organs important for glucose regulation: brain, heart/lungs, gut, liver, kidney, and periphery. The model also includes glucagon dynamics and its interactions with the glucose–insulin system, and consists of 19 ordinary differential equations. The original model was proposed to represent glucose dynamics of a healthy person. However, by removing the equations that describe insulin release, the model can be applied to people with T1D.

A similar physiological model has been proposed by Puckett (1992) to describe glucose–insulin dynamics in a typical person with T1D. The model is developed from patient data except the interstitial insulin transport submodel. The data are collected from people with T1D taking both short- and long-acting insulin. The absorption rate of long-acting insulin is approximated as a zeroth-order process with constant rate. The absorption of regular insulin from the subcutaneous tissue is represented with a two-compartment model. Insulin-independent glucose uptake (glucose uptake by nervous system) rate is assumed constant. Glucose-dependent glucose utilization is assumed to occur only in kidneys where glucose is excreted if the BGC exceeds a limit of 176 mg/dl. Glucosim (Eren et al. 2005; Agar et al. 2006) was developed as an extension of Puckett et al. (1992) model and included 21 ordinary differential equations based on eight different compartments (organs).

The first generation of simulators for glucose–insulin dynamics (Eren et al. 2005; Agar et al. 2006; Hovorka et al. 2004; Reed and Lehmann 2005) used an "average person" with T1D and adjusted some parameters based on personal information of the simulated "person" such as weight and activities such as exercise. They were appropriate for training and education by showing general trends. Recently, the first FDA-approved multipatient UVa/Padova (Kovatchev et al. 2008) metabolic simulator was developed to provide the intra-subject variability. The full version of the simu-

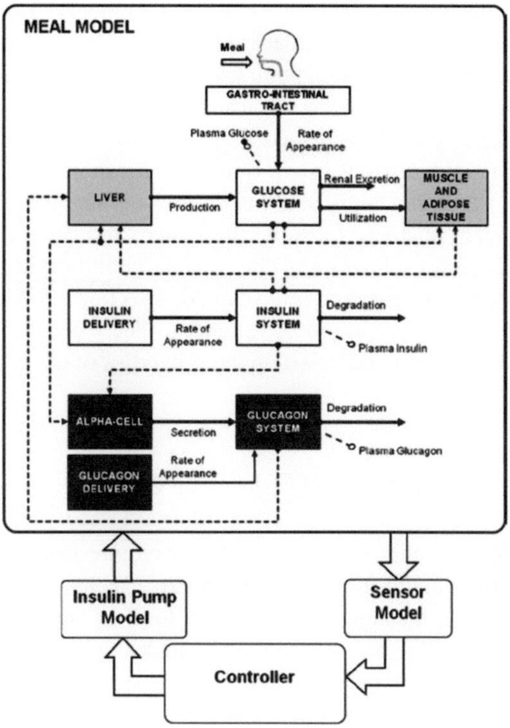

Fig. 4.3 UVa/Padova Glucose/Insulin model. Republished with permission of Sage Publications, from Dalla Man et al. (2014)

lator contains 300 (100 adolescents, 100 adults, and 100 children) virtual patients, and the academic version has ten virtual subjects for each subgroup. The model used in the simulator is highly nonlinear, and the subject-specific model parameters are defined based on clinical data. A newer version of UVa/Padova simulator was proposed Dalla Man et al. (2014) where the glucose dynamics are redefined during hypoglycemic episodes and glucagon kinetics are added with extra compartments (Fig. 4.3).

4.2 Time Series Models and System Identification

Most physical, chemical, and biological systems can be modeled based on mass, energy, and momentum balance equations by using first principles. These models require detailed knowledge about the system, expressed as differential and algebraic equations and logical relations. However, many biological systems are too complex to fully understand or to develop detailed first-principles models that describe their dynamical behavior. Input–output models expressed as time series models, and state-space models provide the ability to express how the inputs of a system affect the behavior of its outputs. Input–output models trade off ease and speed of model development for detailed description of the internal mechanisms of the system that can only be represented by first-principles models. Time series models (and their equivalents in state space) are usually low order and less complex, and they are identified based on data collected by perturbing the inputs and recording the corresponding output variations in the system (Söderström and Stoica 1988).

System identification to develop a time series model requires decisions on experiment planning to excite the system and collect data that represent many possible dynamic behaviors of the system, definition of performance criteria to assess the quality of the model developed, selection of model structure, estimation of model parameters, and model validation. These decisions are system-specific and are usually determined based on the properties of the system to be modeled.

4.2.1 Experiment Planning for Data Collection

Identification methods that do not require special inputs are preferred since it is often costly and difficult to conduct experiments to collect data. Many classical methods depend on input signals in the form of step, gate, impulse, or sinusoid functions while more recent techniques can deal with any type of input signals, at the expense of increased computation cost. A good input signal should excite all the modes of a system to enable the development of an input–output model that can represent the behavior of the system for many types of input changes.

4.2.2 Selection of Model Structure

Prior knowledge about a system and the disturbance(s) to be modeled is used for selecting a suitable model structure. Optimization of the model structure is usually integrated with the computation of the optimal model parameters. Selection of nonlinear model structures necessitates knowledge about the nonlinearities of the system. Fortunately, many systems that operate in the vicinity of an operating point can be described by linear models. Two options are considered if the system operates in regions that change over time: linear models with time-varying parameters and recursive models where the model parameters are updated when new data are received. Several standard time series model structures are summarized below.

Autoregressive eXogenous (ARX) Model: The ARX model expresses the model output at sample time k as a weighted sum of earlier outputs and inputs ($u(k)$) and a white disturbance (noise) term ($\varepsilon(k)$) (Fig. 4.4):

$$y(k) + a_1 y(k-1) + \cdots + a_{na} y(k-na) = b_1 u(k-1) + \cdots + b_{nb} u(k-nb) + \varepsilon(k) \tag{4.1}$$

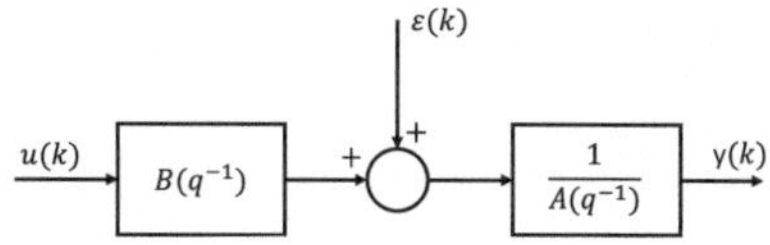

Fig. 4.4 ARX model block diagram

By using the backward shifting operator q^{-1}, the model is expressed as

$$A(q^{-1})y(k) = B(q^{-1})u(k) + \varepsilon(k) \tag{4.2}$$

where the polynomials $A(q^{-1})$ and $B(q^{-1})$ are

$$A(q^{-1}) = 1 + a_1q^{-1} + \cdots + a_{na}q^{-na} \qquad B(q^{-1}) = b_1q^{-1} + \cdots + b_{nb}q^{-nb} \tag{4.3}$$

with na and nb are the positive model orders. Both the input (control) signal and the disturbance are modeled by the same characteristic equation. This type of model is used when the disturbances enter and travel through the system.

Autoregressive Moving Average eXogenous (ARMAX) Model: An ARMAX model (4.4) includes a modeled disturbance

$$A(q^{-1})y(k) = B(q^{-1})u(k) + C(q^{-1})\varepsilon(k) \tag{4.4}$$

where

$$C(q^{-1}) = 1 + c_1q^{-1} + \cdots + c_{nc}q^{-nc} \tag{4.5}$$

The ARMAX model provides more flexibility for modeling disturbances acting on the system that enter at an early stage of the system (close to the input signal), since both the input and disturbances are modeled by the same characteristic polynomial A (Fig. 4.5). The $\varepsilon(k)$ sequence can be substituted by the residuals $e(k)$, the difference between the measured and estimated values of $y(k)$) at past sampling times, to improve the predictions of $y(k)$.

General Model: The general model captures both the individual characteristics of various inputs and the overall dynamics of the system. This model provides flexibility for representing both the system dynamics and stochastic dynamics. The deterministic transfer function (Fig. 4.6) specifies the relationship between the output and the input signals. The stochastic transfer function specifies how the random disturbance

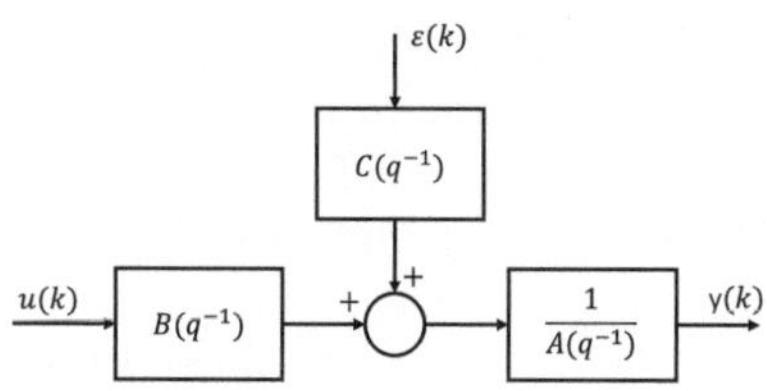

Fig. 4.5 ARMAX model diagram

Fig. 4.6 General model block diagram

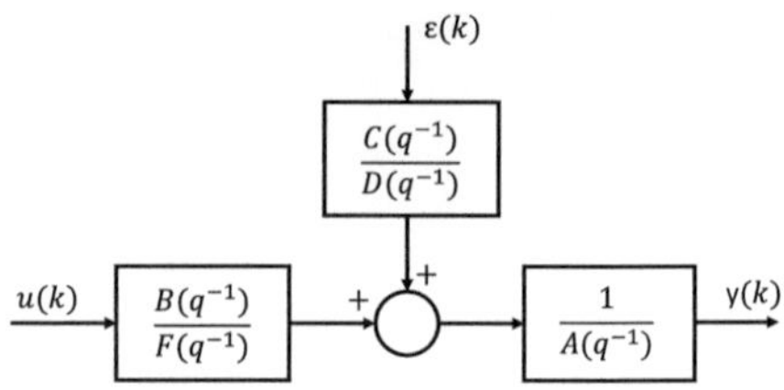

$\varepsilon(k)$ affects the output signal. Often the deterministic and stochastic parts of a system are referred to as system dynamics and stochastic dynamics, respectively.

$$A(q^{-1})y(k) = \frac{B(q^{-1})}{F(q^{-1})}u(k) + \frac{C(q^{-1})}{D(q^{-1})}\varepsilon(k) \tag{4.6}$$

where

$$D(q^{-1}) = 1 + d_1q^{-1} + \cdots + d_{nd}q^{-nd} \quad F(q^{-1}) = 1 + f_1q^{-1} + \cdots + f_{nf}q^{-nf} \tag{4.7}$$

Output Error (OE) Model: The OE model can be used when disturbances mainly influence the measurements of the output signal (such as sensor noise):

$$y(k) = \frac{B(q^{-1})}{F(q^{-1})}u(k) + \varepsilon(k) \tag{4.8}$$

The dynamics caused by changes in the input are identified by the OE model but the dynamics caused by disturbances are neglected. The OE model can be represented by Fig. 4.6 where polynomials A, C, D are set to unity.

Box-Jenkins (BJ) Model: BJ model is usable when the input signal and the disturbances have different dynamic characteristics.

$$y(k) = \frac{B(q^{-1})}{F(q^{-1})}u(k) + \frac{C(q^{-1})}{D(q^{-1})}\varepsilon(k) \tag{4.9}$$

The model provides completely independent parameterization for the dynamics and the disturbances using rational polynomial functions. The deterministic and stochastic parts of the system are identified independently. The BJ model can be represented by Fig. 4.6 where polynomial A is set to unity.

Multivariable Models. All models introduced so far represented systems with single-input single-output (SISO). However, these model structures can be extended to multi-input multi-output (MIMO) formats. For example, a MIMO system is described by an ARX model as

$$\boldsymbol{A}(q^{-1})\boldsymbol{y}(k) = \boldsymbol{B}(q^{-1})\boldsymbol{u}(k) + \boldsymbol{\varepsilon}(k) \tag{4.10}$$

$$\boldsymbol{A}(q^{-1}) = I + A_1 q^{-1} + \cdots + A_{na} q^{-na} \tag{4.11}$$

$$\boldsymbol{B}(q^{-1}) = B_1 q^{-1} + \cdots + B_{nb} q^{-nb} \tag{4.12}$$

where $\boldsymbol{y}(k)$ and $\boldsymbol{u}(k)$ are the output and input vectors with dimensions $ny \times 1$ and $nu \times 1$, respectively. $A_1, \cdots, A_{na}$ are $ny \times ny$ matrices, and $B_1, \cdots, B_{nb}$ are $nu \times nu$ matrices with unknown parameters to be estimated from data.

4.2.3 Model Performance Criteria

Various criteria have been proposed to evaluate how well a model fits the experimental data. A typical criterion for discrete-time system is

$$J(\theta) = \sum_{k=1}^{N} g(e(k)) \tag{4.13}$$

where $e(k)$ is a generalized model error or the residual between the measured process output $y(k)$ and its estimate $\hat{y}(k)$

$$e(k) = y(k) - \hat{y}(k) \tag{4.14}$$

N is the number of data points, and g is usually a quadratic function. The criterion is then used in a parameter estimation method such as least squares (LS) or maximum likelihood (ML) for identification of the unknown model parameters. LS is based on the minimization of the sum of squares of error $e(k)$ and has been used extensively for models that have a linear structure in the unknown parameters.

When the disturbances to a system are described as stochastic processes, model identification can be formulated as a statistical parameter estimation problem. In this framework, the ML method can be considered equivalent to the LS criterion if the quantity to be minimized is taken as the sum of squares of the prediction error. The ML method can be applied to a wide variety of model structures.

4.2.4 Parameter Estimation

Parameter estimation is an optimization problem where model parameters that give the best estimate of the data are identified according to the criterion used. A large number of parameter estimation methods have been proposed depending on experimental conditions, model structures, and criteria used. The estimation methods can be divided into online and off-line parameter estimation. Online methods provide new parameter estimates recursively as new measurements become available. They are used if the process has time-varying dynamics or the model is part of an adaptive controller. Off-line techniques are known to provide more stable parameter estimates when the identified process is time-invariant.

Least Squares Method. A set of parameters is estimated by the LS method such that the difference between the process output and its estimate $\hat{y}(k)$ by the model is minimized. Assume that the process can be described as a linear regression model

$$y(k) = \phi^T(k)\hat{\theta} + \varepsilon(k) \tag{4.15}$$

where ϕ is the vector of regressor variables

$$\phi^T(k) = \left[-y(k-1) \cdots -y(k-na)\; u(k-1) \cdots u(k-nb)\right] \tag{4.16}$$

$\hat{\theta}$ is the vector of parameters that are estimated

$$\hat{\theta} = \left[a_1 \cdots a_{na}\; b_1 \cdots b_{nb}\right]^T \tag{4.17}$$

The LS method estimates the unknown model parameters by minimizing the loss function $V_N(\hat{\theta})$ (Eq. 4.18) that depends on N and $\hat{\theta}$:

$$V_N(\hat{\theta}) = \sum_{k=1}^{N} e(k)^2 \tag{4.18}$$

The minimum of Eq. 4.18 is computed by setting the partial derivative to zero:

$$\frac{\partial V_N(\hat{\theta})}{\partial \hat{\theta}} = 0 \tag{4.19}$$

An analytical solution for estimating $\hat{\theta}$ is obtained by inserting Eqs. 4.14 and 4.15 into Eq. 4.18 and setting its partial derivative to 0, yielding:

$$\hat{\theta} = \left[\sum_{k=1}^{N} \phi(k)\phi^T(k)\right]^{-1} \left[\sum_{k=1}^{N} \phi(k)y(k)\right] \tag{4.20}$$

Pseudo Least Squares Method. The LS method gives biased estimates when the disturbances $\varepsilon(k)$ acting on the system are correlated with the regressor $\phi(k)$. This happens when $\varepsilon(k)$ is not white noise and is considered as colored noise. Bias in estimations means that the parameter values are systematically different from their actual values. One way to handle colored noise is to incorporate a noise term to model. For example, ARMAX models have a term related to noise, but the numerical values of the noise term in ARMAX model are not known. The pseudo LS method deals with this problem by considering the residuals (Eq. 4.14) as white noise. The linear regression form of the ARMAX model under pseudo LS is

$$y(k) = \phi^T(k)\hat{\theta} + e(k) \tag{4.21}$$

$$\begin{aligned}\phi^T(k) = [&-y(k-1)\cdots - y(k-na)\ \ u(k-1)\cdots u(k-nb) \\ &e(k-1)\cdots e(k-nc)]\end{aligned} \tag{4.22}$$

$$\hat{\theta} = \begin{bmatrix} a_1 & \cdots & a_{na} & b_1 \cdots & b_{nb} & c_1 & \cdots & c_{nc} \end{bmatrix}^T \tag{4.23}$$

Instrumental Variable Method. The IV method is another way to handle bias in estimated parameters when ARX model is preferred. The IV method transforms the residuals (Eq. 4.14) with matrix $Z(k)$ such that the colored noise characteristics disappear. This is obtained by solving

$$\frac{1}{N}\sum_{k=1}^{N} Z(k)e(k) = \frac{1}{N}\sum_{k=1}^{N} Z(k)\left[y(k) - \phi^T(k)\hat{\theta}\right] = 0 \tag{4.24}$$

An analytical solution for parameter estimation with the basic IV method is

$$\hat{\theta} = \left[\sum_{k=1}^{N} Z(k)\phi^T(k)\right]^{-1}\left[\sum_{k=1}^{N} Z(k)y(k)\right] \tag{4.25}$$

where the dimensions of $Z(k)$ are $n_{\hat{\theta}} \times n_y$. $Z(k)$ can be defined by using various algorithms (Nelles 2013).

Maximum Likelihood Method. When the disturbances acting on the process are uncorrelated noise with Normal distribution, the distribution of the residuals follows the same distribution as the disturbances. The probability distribution of the residuals $e(k)$ based on the parameters vector $\hat{\theta}$ is

$$P\left[e(k)|\hat{\theta}\right] = \frac{1}{\sqrt{2\pi}\sigma(\hat{\theta})} exp\left(\frac{e^2(k,\hat{\theta})}{2\sigma^2(\hat{\theta})}\right) \tag{4.26}$$

where σ represent the standard deviation. Since the residuals are assumed to be independent, the likelihood function is formulated as the product of the probability function of each sample. The optimal parameters are estimated by maximizing the likelihood function $L(\hat{\theta})$

$$L(\hat{\theta}) = P\left[e(1)|\hat{\theta}\right]\cdot \ldots \cdot P\left[e(N)|\hat{\theta}\right] \tag{4.27}$$

Substitution of Eqs. 4.26 into 4.27 gives:

$$L(\hat{\theta}) = \frac{1}{\left[\sqrt{2\pi}\sigma(\hat{\theta})\right]^N} exp\left(\sum_{k=1}^{N} \frac{e^2(k,\hat{\theta})}{2\sigma^2(\hat{\theta})}\right) \tag{4.28}$$

It is practical to take the natural logarithm of $L(\hat{\theta})$ and convert it to a minimization problem

$$log(L(\hat{\theta})) = \sum_{k=1}^{N} \frac{e^2(k,\hat{\theta})}{2\sigma^2(\hat{\theta})} - \frac{N}{2} log(2\pi\sigma^2(\hat{\theta})) \tag{4.29}$$

The ML method can be extended to MIMO systems. Let the covariance matrix of the residuals be R_σ. The likelihood and log likelihood functions become

$$L(\hat{\theta}) = \frac{1}{\left[\sqrt{2\pi}\right]^{n_y N/2} [det R_\sigma]^{N/2}} exp\left(\frac{1}{2}\sum_{k=1}^{N} e^T(k,\hat{\theta}) R_\sigma^{-1} e(k,\hat{\theta})\right) \tag{4.30}$$

$$log(L(\hat{\theta})) = \sum_{k=1}^{N} e^T(k,\hat{\theta}) R_\sigma^{-1} e(k,\hat{\theta}) - \frac{N}{2} log(det\ R_\sigma) + constant \tag{4.31}$$

When $R_\sigma = \sigma^2 I$, Eq. 4.31 is equivalent to the LS method.

Numerical Minimization of the Loss Function. Finding the minimum of $V_N(\hat{\theta})$ involves complicated computations. Unlike the LS method, most of the identification methods do not have an analytical solution and require numerical methods to solve the minimization problem. A simple method to numerically find the minimum is to iterate on the unknown parameters. The loss function $V_N(\hat{\theta}_1)$ is computed with an initial value of parameters $\hat{\theta}_1$. Then, the parameters are changed in the direction where $V_N(\hat{\theta}_1)$ decreases. The iterations are repeated until the minimum of $V_N(\hat{\theta}_1)$ is achieved. The Newton–Raphson method is a popular method for finding iteratively the optimal parameter values

$$\hat{\theta}^{i+1} = \hat{\theta}^i - \gamma_i \frac{V_N'(\hat{\theta})}{V_N''(\hat{\theta})} \tag{4.32}$$

where γ is the step length and $V_N'(\hat{\theta})$ and $V_N''(\hat{\theta})$ are the first and second derivatives of the loss function, respectively.

4.2.5 Model Analysis

When a model is derived from experimental data, it is necessary to validate the model with data not used in model development. Techniques such as cross-validation provide a systematic procedure for model validation.

Simulation and Prediction. The model developed can be utilized for simulation and prediction by using the inputs given to the system. The model outputs are compared with data from experiments. In simulation, a good match between the current measured and estimated outputs is sought. In prediction, a match between future values of data (obtained from historical databases) and estimated values is compared during model (estimator) development. The system output is predicted j time steps ahead of the current time, by using process information up to the present time k ($\hat{y}(j+k|k)$). Good prediction capability is critical for a model that will be used in model-based control systems. The dynamics of the measured and estimated outputs should be similar (Fig. 4.7). In general, the j-steps-ahead predictions have larger deviations from system data as j increases.

When a model is identified using different experimental datasets from the same process, the estimated parameters might be slightly different from each other depending on different dynamic system behaviors captured in various datasets. This becomes more acute if the physical system is nonlinear or has time-varying parameters. Usually the mean of the corresponding standard deviation is used as the final parameter estimation. However, it is still important to check how the model output behaves with all uncertain parameter estimates. An example of model simulation for uncertainty in parameter estimation is shown in Fig. 4.8. Based on the standard deviation, the values of the estimated parameters are chosen randomly and the model is tested with a step input.

Statistical Analysis. The residual (innovation) sequence $e(k)$ is used to analyze the lack of fit between the model and system outputs. The residuals contain information about unmodeled system dynamics or disturbances. When the model is an accurate representation of the system, the residuals sequence is zero-mean white noise with Normal distribution. White noise residuals have no correlation between sequences or with any other system signals. In other words, there is no information left in the residuals that could improve the model. A simple inspection of the residuals is to

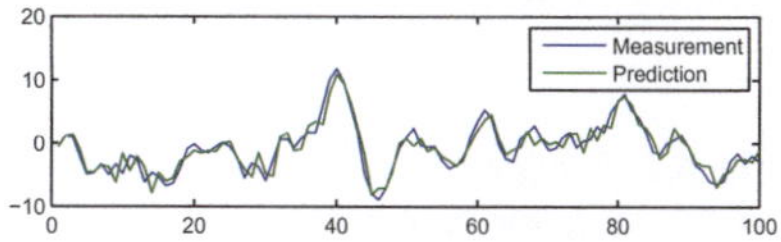

Fig. 4.7 Comparison of experimental and 1-step-ahead predicted outputs

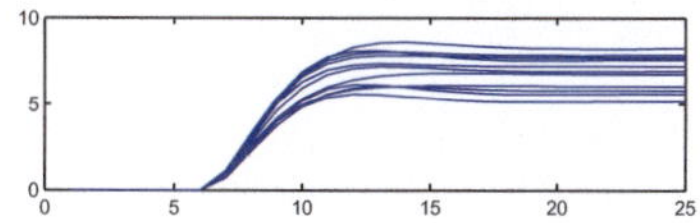

Fig. 4.8 Simulation with uncertainties in estimated model parameters

plot them on a time diagram. Trends in the plot with peaks and nadirs without any significant pattern are indicative of white noise. If there is a periodicity or patterns in the residuals, they cannot be considered to be white noise.

Various criteria are used to check if the residual sequence is white noise, including the autocorrelation of the residuals, the cross-correlation between the residual and input signals, and the distribution of the residuals. The statistical tests are based on the null hypotheses that:

1. The residuals are zero-mean white noise.
2. The residuals have a symmetric distribution.
3. The residuals have Normal distribution.
4. The residuals are independent of each other.
5. The residuals are independent of all other signals.

The autocorrelation of the residuals is computed as

$$r_{auto}(\tau) = \frac{1}{N-\tau}\sum_{k=1}^{N-\tau} e(k)e(k+\tau) \tag{4.33}$$

where τ is a nonnegative parameter and represents the lag between samples. When $\tau = 0$, Eq. 4.33 represents the variance of the residual sequence. A useful way to analyze the autocorrelation is to plot the autocorrelation as a function of the lag τ. The diagram is extended with 99% confidence interval defined as $(-2.58/\sqrt{N}, 2.58/\sqrt{N})$ where N is the number of data points.

The dependence between the residuals and inputs, cross-correlation, is tested similarly

$$r_{cross}(\tau) = \frac{1}{N-\tau}\sum_{k=1}^{N-\tau} e(k+\tau)u(k) \tag{4.34}$$

The cross-correlation test is made for both positive and negative values of τ. Cross-correlation is compared with the 99% confidence interval as well. A peak in negative or positive side of the cross-correlation indicates a feedback or a time delay in the process that is not been incorporated in the model, respectively (Fig. 4.9).

Another residual test is performed by comparing the histogram of residuals with the corresponding Normal distribution to determine whether the residuals have Normal distribution.

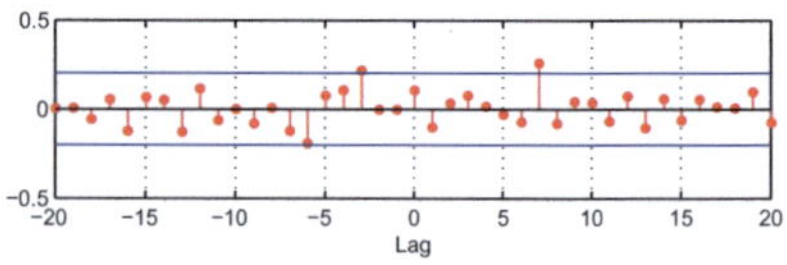

Fig. 4.9 Sample cross-correlation function. Feedback at lag −3 and delay at lag 7

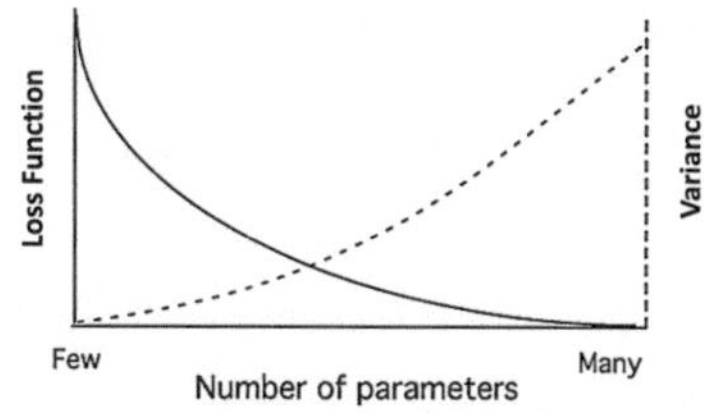

Fig. 4.10 Loss function versus variance

Model Structure Analysis. A good model has small residuals. Loss (cost) function can be used as a measure of model accuracy. When the number model parameters increases, the loss function is reduced (Fig. 4.10, solid line). However, a model with too many parameters may be overdetermined. The increase in the number of parameters will increase the variance of the estimated values (Fig. 4.10, dashed line). Consequently, more parameters will create problems with reproducibility of the parameters. One way to deal with this problem is to introduce a criterion that balances the magnitude of the loss function and the number of estimated parameters. Some popular criteria include:

Akaike's Information Criterion (AIC)

$$V_{AIC} = \left(1 + 2\frac{d}{N}\right)\frac{1}{N}\sum_{k=1}^{N} e^2(k) \tag{4.35}$$

Rissanen's Minimum Description Length Criterion (MDL)

$$V_{MDL} = \left(1 + \log(N)\frac{d}{N}\right)\frac{1}{N}\sum_{k=1}^{N} e^2(k) \tag{4.36}$$

Final Prediction Error (FPE)

$$V_{FPE} = \frac{1 + \frac{d}{N}}{1 - \frac{d}{N}}\frac{1}{N}\sum_{k=1}^{N} e^2(k) \tag{4.37}$$

where d is the number parameters and N is the number of samples.

Parameter Analysis. When the values of some estimated parameters are close to zero within the limits of the standard deviation, the estimated parameters can be neglected. The pole–zero diagram can be used to analyze overdetermination of the model in which case some poles or zeros are located within uncertainty intervals of others. The pole–zero diagram on the right side of Fig. 4.11 illustrates the overlap of the uncertainty intervals of some poles and zeros. The overlapped poles and zeros are cancelling their effects. The model order should be decreased in order to eliminate overlapping of poles and zeros.

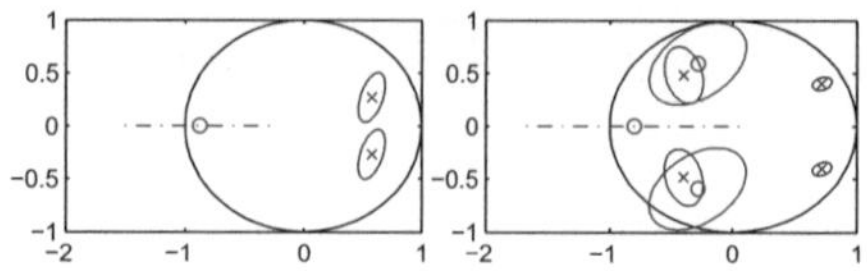

Fig. 4.11 Pole–Zero diagram (Left). Pole–Zero cancellation (Right). (x:poles, o:zeros)

Frequency Analysis. Frequency analysis indicates if the model is able to capture the frequency relation between the input and output of the system. The input signal should be chosen such that the interested frequency interval is excited.

The frequency characteristics of a measured signal are estimated by using Fourier analysis. Let $\Phi_u(w)$ and $\Phi_{yu}(w)$ be the input spectrum and cross-spectrum between input and output signals, respectively. The process transfer function between the input and output is:

$$\hat{G}(jw) = \frac{\hat{\Phi}_{yu}(w)}{\hat{\Phi}_u(w)} \tag{4.38}$$

$$\hat{\Phi}_{yu}(w) = \sum_{\tau=-\gamma}^{\gamma} \hat{R}_{yu}(\tau)e^{-\tau \cdot jw} \quad \hat{R}_{yu}(\tau) = \frac{1}{N}\sum_{k=1}^{N-\tau} y(k+\tau)u(k) \tag{4.39}$$

$$\hat{\Phi}_{u}(w) = \sum_{\tau=-\gamma}^{\gamma} \hat{R}_{u}(\tau)e^{-\tau \cdot jw} \quad \hat{R}_{u}(\tau) = \frac{1}{N}\sum_{k=1}^{N-\tau} u(k+\tau)u(k) \tag{4.40}$$

4.3 Recursive Time Series Models

Most complex systems can be represented by models with time-varying parameters. For such systems, a model that has been identified based on a specific operating (stationary) point may not be able to track the process behavior at another operating point due to dynamic changes in system characteristics overtime. Thus, it is necessary to update or adapt some or all model parameters in real time to reproduce the actual behavior of the system. Modeling techniques where parameter estimates for the current period are calculated by using only recent data and latest parameter estimates are called "recursive" estimation techniques. Updating parameter estimates as new data arrives has considerable computational advantages over the standard practice of re-estimation using the entire (larger) data set. Storage requirements are also reduced as past data need not be retained.

The residuals are the inputs to the parameter update step in recursive estimation. A recursive estimation algorithm based on LS method, also known as recursive least squares (RLS), can be formulated as:

$$\hat{y}(k) = \phi^T(k)\hat{\theta}(k-1) \tag{4.41}$$

$$e(k) = y(k) - \hat{y}(k) \tag{4.42}$$

$$P(k) = P(k-1) - \frac{P(k-1)\phi(k)\phi^T(k)P(k-1)}{1 + \phi^T(k)P(k-1)\phi(k)} \tag{4.43}$$

$$K(k) = P(k)\phi(k) \tag{4.44}$$

$$\hat{\theta}(k) = \hat{\theta}(k-1) + K(k)e(k) \tag{4.45}$$

where the initial conditions can be set as $\hat{\theta}(0) = 0$ and $P(0) = Constant \cdot I$ when there is no knowledge about the parameters. I is the identity matrix.

Recursive estimation is designed to track rapid changes in parameter values and be insensitive to disturbances acting on the system. However, when the estimation is too insensitive to disturbances, the ability to follow fast changes is reduced. One way to address the trade-off between insensitivity to disturbances and fast tracking of dynamical changes in RLS is to use a forgetting factor λ. The forgetting factor enables the latest measurement to have a greater impact on the loss function compared to earlier measurements. The loss function with a forgetting factor is:

$$V_k(\hat{\theta}) = \sum_{i=1}^{k} \lambda^{k-i} e^2(i) \tag{4.46}$$

where $0 < \lambda < 1$. The choice of the λ depends on the desired dynamics of the recursive algorithm and disturbances in measurements. When $\lambda = 1$, the estimator gives equal weight to all data (infinite memory). A small value of λ gives more weight on recent observations (short memory). The estimator is slow and insensitive to disturbances for large values of λ.

When λ is used, the error covariance matrix in Eq. 4.43 becomes:

$$P(k) = \frac{1}{\lambda}\left[P(k-1) - \frac{P(k-1)\phi(k)\phi^T(k)P(k-1)}{\lambda + \phi^T(k)P(k-1)\phi(k)}\right] \tag{4.47}$$

4.4 State-Space Models

State-space models can efficiently describe high-order SISO and MIMO systems. The state-space model contains all the information to predict the behavior of a system at any time t (or k for discrete-time state-space modes), given the initial conditions (at time t_0) and the sequence of inputs. This means that the future outputs can be predicted if future inputs are known, making the state-space models very attractive for use in model-based control systems such as MPC and GPC. State-space models can be developed by using equations based on first-principles and compartmental models or directly from data.

In general, when a system of order n_a is represented with a state-space model, it is necessary to define n_a states. The input, output, and state vectors of a system with n_u inputs and n_y outputs are

$$\boldsymbol{u}(t) = \begin{bmatrix} u_1(t) \\ \cdots \\ u_{nu}(t) \end{bmatrix} \quad \boldsymbol{y}(t) = \begin{bmatrix} y_1(t) \\ \cdots \\ y_{ny}(t) \end{bmatrix} \quad \boldsymbol{x}(t) = \begin{bmatrix} x_1(t) \\ \cdots \\ x_{na}(t) \end{bmatrix} \tag{4.48}$$

The continuous state-space representation is given as:

$$\begin{aligned} \dot{\boldsymbol{x}}(t) &= \boldsymbol{A}\boldsymbol{x}(t) + \boldsymbol{B}\boldsymbol{u}(t) + v(t) \\ \boldsymbol{y}(t) &= \boldsymbol{C}\boldsymbol{x}(t) + \boldsymbol{D}\boldsymbol{u}(t) + w(t) \end{aligned} \tag{4.49}$$

$$\begin{aligned} \boldsymbol{A} &= \begin{bmatrix} a_{1,1} & \cdots & a_{1,na} \\ \cdots & \cdots\cdots & \\ a_{na,1} & \cdots & a_{na,na} \end{bmatrix} \quad \boldsymbol{B} = \begin{bmatrix} b_{1,1} & \cdots & b_{1,nu} \\ \cdots & \cdots\cdots & \\ b_{na,1} & \cdots & a_{na,nu} \end{bmatrix} \\ \boldsymbol{C} &= \begin{bmatrix} c_{1,1} & \cdots & c_{1,na} \\ \cdots & \cdots\cdots & \\ c_{ny,1} & \cdots & c_{ny,na} \end{bmatrix} \quad \boldsymbol{D} = \begin{bmatrix} d_{1,1} & \cdots & d_{1,nu} \\ \cdots & \cdots\cdots & \\ d_{ny,1} & \cdots & d_{ny,nu} \end{bmatrix} \end{aligned} \tag{4.50}$$

where $v(t)$ and $w(t)$ represent process and measurement noise, respectively. The continuous state-space form can be transformed to a corresponding discrete state space model. Denoting the state vector at sampling time t_k as $x(k)$ and the input vector during the sampling interval is $u(k)$, the state vector at sampling time t_{k+1} is denoted by $x(k+1)$ and is expressed by the solution of the continuous state-space model as:

$$\begin{aligned} \boldsymbol{x}(k+1) &= e^{\boldsymbol{A}(t_{k+1}-t_k)}\boldsymbol{x}(k) + \int_{t_k}^{t_{k+1}} e^{\boldsymbol{A}(t_{k+1}-t)}\boldsymbol{B}\boldsymbol{u}(k)dt + v(k) \\ \boldsymbol{y}(k) &= \boldsymbol{C}\boldsymbol{x}(k) + \boldsymbol{D}\boldsymbol{u}(k) + w(k) \end{aligned} \tag{4.51}$$

where the time at the sample instances is given by $t_k = k \cdot h$ and h is the sampling time which is used to derive a compact discrete state-space model form:

$$\begin{aligned} \boldsymbol{x}(k+1) &= \boldsymbol{F}\boldsymbol{x}(k) + \boldsymbol{G}\boldsymbol{u}(k) + v(k) \\ \boldsymbol{y}(k) &= \boldsymbol{C}\boldsymbol{x}(k) + \boldsymbol{D}\boldsymbol{u}(k) + w(k) \end{aligned} \tag{4.52}$$

where

$$\boldsymbol{F} = e^{\boldsymbol{A}h} \quad \boldsymbol{G} = \int_0^h e^{\boldsymbol{A}t}dt\, \boldsymbol{B} \tag{4.53}$$

Chapter 5
Alarm Systems

Abstract Alarm systems warn people with T1D when hypoglycemia occurs or can be predicted to occur in the near future if the current glucose concentration trends continue. Various alarm system development strategies are outlined in this chapter. Severe hypoglycemia has significant effects ranging from dizziness to diabetic coma and death while long periods of hyperglycemia cause damage to the vascular system. Fear of hypoglycemia is a major concern for many people with T1D. High doses of exogenous insulin relative to food, activity and low blood glucose levels can precipitate hypoglycemia. Hypoglycemia and hyperglycemia early alarm systems would be very beneficial for people with T1D to warn them or their caregivers about the potential hypoglycemia and hyperglycemia episode before it happens and empowers them to take measures to prevent these events.

Keywords Hypoglycemia · Hyperglycemia · Alarms · Predictive alarms

The goal of new therapeutic options for people with T1D is to increase the time spent in euglycemia without increasing the risk of hypoglycemia. However, tight glycemic control is achieved by an aggressive controller, which increases the risk for severe hypoglycemia. Intensive insulin treatment improves glycemic control, but it can increase the risk for severe hypoglycemia compared to conventional treatment, resulting in a higher incidence of complications (National Institute of Diabetes and Digestive and Kidney Diseases 2016). In all adolescent Diabetes Control and Complications Trial participants, intensive treatment of T1D increased the frequency of severe hypoglycemia from two to six times that observed with conventional treatment (National Institute of Diabetes and Digestive and Kidney Diseases 2016). Another risk factor for severe hypoglycemia is hypoglycemia unawareness, which occurs in about 10% of patients and prevents them from recognizing and treating symptoms of hypoglycemia (National Institute of Diabetes and Digestive and Kidney Diseases 2016). More than 50% of severe hypoglycemic episodes occur during sleep, and sudden nocturnal death due to nocturnal hypoglycemia in young people with T1D

A. Cinar and K. Turksoy, *Advances in Artificial Pancreas Systems*,
SpringerBriefs in Bioengineering, https://doi.org/10.1007/978-3-319-72245-0_5

is responsible for about 6% of deaths in people with T1D younger than 40 years of age (National Institute of Diabetes and Digestive and Kidney Diseases 2016).

People with T1D trying to improve or maintain glucose control may experience asymptomatic hypoglycemia up to 10% of the time (Cryer et al. 2003). They experience on average two episodes of symptomatic hypoglycemia per week and one episode of severe hypoglycemia per year (Cryer et al. 2003). About 2–4% of deaths of people with T1D are attributed to hypoglycemia (Cryer et al. 2003). From 2001 to 2010, the average annual number of hospitalizations for adults aged 18 years and older attributed to hypoglycemia was 285,800 (National Institute of Diabetes and Digestive and Kidney Diseases 2016). The number of emergency room visits for hypoglycemia for adults aged 18 years and older stayed stable between 2006 and 2009, with about 298,000 visits in 2009, while the number of visits for hyperglycemic crisis for all ages increased from 150,000 to 170,000 during the same period (Centers for Disease Control and Prevention 2014, 2012). In 2011, about 282,000 emergency room visits for adults aged 18 years and older were attributed to hypoglycemia, and about 175,000 were attributed to hyperglycemic crisis such as diabetic ketoacidosis or hyperglycemic hyperosmolar state (Centers for Disease Control and Prevention and Others 2014).

Although the goal of the AP is to optimize glycemic control and reduce the burden on the patient via a closed-loop system, maintaining the safety of the user may sometimes require open-loop intervention to prevent hypoglycemia. One of the concerns with closed-loop systems is the possibility that the system will not recognize a hypoglycemic event or conditions that will lead to such an event and will continue to infuse insulin, causing a great danger to the user (Skladnev et al. 2010). One way to improve the safety of these systems is to incorporate hypoglycemia alarm algorithms that predict hypoglycemia and prevent it, either by automated means such as insulin pump suspension or by alerting the user and initiating open-loop intervention such as alerts for consumption of rescue CHOs. Some CGM devices and insulin pumps incorporate alarms based on current CGM readings or BGC predictions.

Many studies have been done to assess the ability of different hypoglycemia alarm systems to predict hypoglycemia. Algorithms used in these hypoglycemia alarm systems have utilized only CGM data (Palerm and Bequette 2007; Eren-Oruklu et al. 2009, 2010; Buckingham et al. 2009; Dassau et al. 2010; Bayrak et al. 2012; Gani et al. 2009; Reifman et al. 2007, or CGM and insulin pump data Hughes et al. 2010), or CGM and insulin pump data along with physiological variable data (Turksoy et al. 2013c).

Incorporating physiological response data improved the sensitivity of the alarm algorithm by 10% for the same specificity, meaning that the number of missed hypoglycemic events was reduced while the number of false positives remained the same (Skladnev et al. 2010). Subject-specific recursive linear time series models (Turksoy et al. 2013c; Eren-Oruklu et al. 2009, 2010) were used in some studies because they enabled dynamic adaptation of the models to inter-/intra-subject variations and glycemic disturbances. Kalman filters were used in one algorithm to obtain the most likely estimate of glucose concentration and its first and second derivatives by trading off the probability that a measured glucose change is due to sensor noise rather than actual change in glucose levels (Palerm and Bequette 2007). Recursive autoregressive partial least squares models were used in another study to predict future BGC. This method improves upon traditional partial least squares models by including autoregressive terms to capture dynamic changes in glucose data as well as by using recursive updates to remove the influence of old data (Bayrak et al. 2012). Other hypoglycemia prediction methods include linear prediction, statistical prediction, adaptive hybrid infinite impulse response (HIIR) filtering, and numerical logical algorithms. These algorithms, along with Kalman filtering, were used in a voting system to improve decision accuracy. Concurrent use of multiple algorithms improves safety and prevents the user from relying on a single algorithm that may not be the most suitable to accommodate glucose variability (Buckingham et al. 2009; Dassau et al. 2010). In these studies, critical algorithm parameters such as hypoglycemia threshold and prediction horizon were selected based on performance, the goal being to maximize hypoglycemia detection within enough time to provide effective intervention while minimizing the number of false alarms.

Even though hypoglycemia alarm systems would be very helpful in improving safety and mitigating hypoglycemia, some challenges must be addressed to enhance their ability to prevent hypoglycemia. Many hypoglycemic events occur at night, so the potential exists for an alarm to sound while the patient is asleep and cannot react to it, or may not have the means to mitigate it (such as access to oral CHOs). Hence, predicting and preventing hypoglycemia are two different issues. While the algorithm may be able to predict hypoglycemia, action needs to be taken to mitigate or avoid hypoglycemia. Future work should be done to investigate the inclusion of these alarms in fully automated APs to prevent hypoglycemia without requiring user intervention, through a combination of automatic pump suspension and/or glucagon infusion.

Various studies have shown that some hypoglycemia episodes can be prevented by suspension of insulin infusion (Buckingham et al. 2010; Cameron et al. 2012b). However, an AP system with insulin as the only manipulated variable may not be sufficient to prevent all hypoglycemia episodes. When hypoglycemia is detected or predicted, insulin infusion is reduced or suspended and consumption of rescue CHOs may be advised. Several factors influence glycemic response to food, including food form, degree of cooking and processing (particle size, degree of hydration), ripeness, macronutrient composition, fiber, anti-nutrients (e.g., amylase inhibitors), amount of food or CHO consumed at one time, type of sugar (glucose, fructose, sucrose, lactose) or starch (amylose, amylopectin, resistant starch), meal frequency, rate of ingestion, and physiologic effects (Wong and Jenkins 2007; Shils et al. 1998; Franz et al. 2002; Bantle et al. 2008). Any of these factors, alone or in combination, will impact the overall rate of digestion and absorption and subsequent glycemic response. When hypoglycemia is detected, providing a small amount of CHO can help (Franz et al. 2002). Depending on the level BGC and its rate of decrease, providing a rapidly absorbable form of CHO (dextrose tablets or gels, juice, etc.) can quickly increase

BGC levels. Addition of complex CHOs can prevent the hypoglycemia episode from recurring (Shils et al. 1998; Franz et al. 2002).

Glucagon has been used as the second control (manipulated) variable in dual-hormone AP systems to prevent hypoglycemia (El-Khatib et al. 2010; Castle et al. 2010; van Bon et al. 2010; Russell et al. 2012; Van Bon et al. 2012; Haidar et al. 2013; van Bon et al. 2014; Haidar et al. 2014). Glucagon increases glucose by stimulating adenylate cyclase to produce increased cyclic AMP, promoting hepatic glycogenolysis and gluconeogenesis. This antihypoglycemic effect requires preexisting liver glycogen stores (Hegenbarth et al. 2008). Although glucagon works well to prevent low BGC, there have been some occasions where administration of glucagon was not sufficient to fully prevent hypoglycemia and additional rescue CHOs were needed during almost all reported studies. Administration of glucagon can help prevent hypoglycemia if the patient has sufficient glycogen stores, but, if not, then fast-acting CHOs should be provided if the patient is responsive.

Hypoglycemia alarm systems have the potential to improve the safety of AP systems. The studies reported to date show many different algorithms and types of data that could be included in these alarm systems. More extensive testing needs to be done to identify the optimal system. Shorter prediction horizons and higher hypoglycemia thresholds improve hypoglycemia detection, but they also increase the number of false alarms (Eren-Oruklu et al. 2010). These parameters need to be tuned so that the prediction occurs in enough time for intervention to occur and be successful, and the alarm is meaningful to the user (Eren-Oruklu et al. 2010). Some pump systems have added hypoglycemia alarms based on current CGM readings (Medtronic MiniMed 530G). More recent pump development focused on using predictive hypoglycemia alarms (Medtronic MiniMed 640G, Tandem), following the original JDRF road map.

Chapter 6
Various Control Philosophies for AP Systems

Abstract In AP systems, the control algorithm is responsible for calculating the best estimate of basal and bolus insulin and/or glucagon dose based on the patient's glucose concentration estimates and physiological properties, to reach the target glucose range. Various types of control algorithms that have been investigated for AP systems with simulations and clinical experiments over the last three decades are presented. Mathematical details are given for each type of control algorithm and their advantages and limitations are discussed.

Keywords Propotional-Integral-Derivative control · Model predictive control
Generalized predictive control · Knowledge based fuzzy logic control
Adaptive control

The core of the AP is the control algorithm, which uses sensor data to compute insulin dosing instructions for the pump. It calculates the optimal insulin dose based on the patient BGC estimates and physiological properties. In the last three decades various types of control algorithms have been investigated with simulations and clinical animal and human experiments. Clinical experiments showed that proportional-integral-derivative (PID), model predictive control (MPC), generalized predictive control (GPC, adaptive control), and fuzzy logic knowledge-based control systems are promising for BGC regulation.

6.1 Proportional–Integral–Derivative Control

The PID algorithm has been utilized in process industries for the past 80 years. It uses the difference between the reference (set point) and the process output value to generate an error signal $e(t)$ that becomes the input signal to the controller. The PID controller has three elements, also called actions: proportional (P), integral (I), and derivative (D) action. These can be combined in different ways to develop different

A. Cinar and K. Turksoy, *Advances in Artificial Pancreas Systems*,
SpringerBriefs in Bioengineering, https://doi.org/10.1007/978-3-319-72245-0_6

controllers such as P-, PI-, PD- or PID controller. The PID algorithm is the sum of three terms (control actions):

$$u(t) = K_P e(t) + K_I \int_0^t e(t)dt + K_D \frac{de(t)}{dt} \tag{6.1}$$

where K_P, K_I and K_D are the tuning parameters of the controller. Several methods have been proposed to estimate the parameters of the PID controller (Åström and Hägglund 2006; Seborg et al. 2010; Romagnoli and Palazoglu 2005; Ogunnaike 1994). The proportional gain K_P determines the magnitude of the instantaneous response of the controller to the error signal. Larger values of K_P increase the magnitude of the control signal and speed up the response of the system. Large K_P values also reduce the offset between the set point and final steady-state value of the output signal. However, large values of K_P magnify the effect of measurement noise and model uncertainties and may cause instability of the system. The integral action with parameter K_I sums the error values over time to force the steady-state error to zero. The derivative term with parameter K_D responds to directions and magnitudes of change in outputs. Increasing K_D causes the system to react more swiftly to changes in the error and increases the speed of the overall system response. However, large K_D may cause instability, since the derivative term is very sensitive to disturbances and measurement noise. The performance of the PID controller or its sub-combinations is improved by tuning the parameters of controller.

The classical PID control uses only the current value of the error $e(t)$ to compute the control action. Yet, additional information and algorithms can enhance its performance. The shortcomings of PID control are addressed by adding feedforward action for measured disturbances, gain scheduling to adjust the controller gain K_P depending on the magnitude of the error $e(t)$ to reduce overshoots while making rapid changes when large errors are present, and cascade control to enhance the response speed and prevent the effects of some disturbances from reaching the output (Seborg et al. 2010; Romagnoli and Palazoglu 2005; Ogunnaike 1994).

The classical PID has severe handicaps in regulating BGC with an AP. Use of estimates of future BGC values and constraints on maximum changes in insulin infusion rates can improve PID controller performance. Several additional features such as glucose estimators have been proposed to develop a comprehensive AP controller (Steil and Rebrin 2008; Steil et al. 2011; Palerm 2011; Steil 2013).

6.2 Model Predictive Control

To formulate an optimal control problem for a dynamic system, a process model with specified physical limits and a well-defined performance measure is required. An elegant mathematical solution to model-based optimal control problem was presented by Pontryagin (1987), later called the Pontryagin minimum principle. An improve-

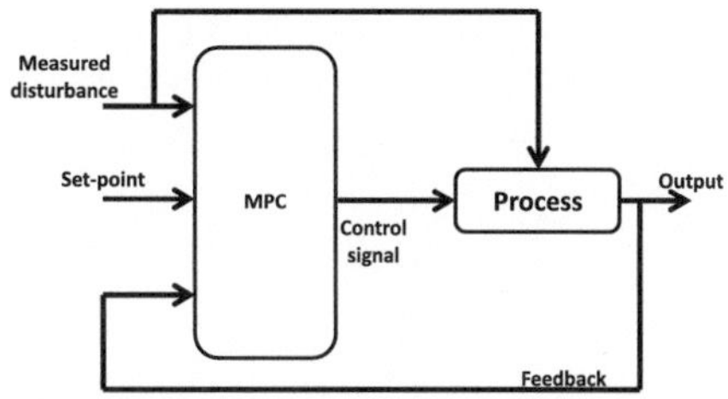

Fig. 6.1 MPC block diagram

ment to make the control problem more realistic was to introduce physical limits on the control signals and process state variables at the same time. The approach leads to a nonlinear two-point boundary problem with a large computation load.

MPC is closely related to the optimal control problem, and the control action is determined by real-time optimization. MPC has two prediction horizons, one for predicting the future values of the controlled variables (process outputs) and the other for changing future settings of manipulated variables (control actions). A performance measure is defined based on the deviations of future process outputs from the desired future reference trajectory and on the magnitude of future control actions. The MPC (Fig. 6.1) is based on four main components:

- A model for predicting the future behavior of process output(s),
- An objective function for optimizing the behavior of the system under MPC,
- An optimization algorithm,
- Constraints on inputs, outputs and their rates of change.

An optimal sequence of future control actions is computed over the control horizon by minimizing an objective function. This is an iterative process where a future control action sequence for the control horizon is hypothesized to initiate the optimization and a constrained optimization is conducted in real time by estimating the future outputs over the prediction horizon, and modifying them during the course of the optimization to determine the optimal sequence of control actions. The control horizon cannot be larger the prediction horizon. Only the first control action (the next time step) is implemented to control the process. Then, the horizon windows are shifted to the next sampling time and the optimization is repeated when the new values of the outputs are measured.

Consider a system described by a discrete state-space model (Eq. 6.2). It is assumed that all states are measurable, and the future of the process states are calculated based on current measurements using the model (6.2)

$$\begin{aligned} x(k+1) &= Fx(k) + Gu(k) + v(k) \\ y(k) &= Cx(k) + w(k) \end{aligned} \tag{6.2}$$

where the states and measurements are affected by white noises $v(k)$ and $w(k)$, respectively, with covariances R_1 and R_2:

Let the $r(k)$ sequence in the prediction horizon be a constant or time-varying future reference trajectory. A quadratic objective function formulates the MPC control law:

$$V = \sum_{j=1}^{N_y} \left|\left|r(k+j) - \hat{y}(k+j)\right|\right|_{Q_1}^2 + \sum_{j=1}^{N_u} ||\Delta u(k+j-1)||_{Q_2}^2 \tag{6.3}$$

where $\left|\left|r(k+j) - \hat{y}(k+j)\right|\right|_{Q_1}^2$ is the short notation for the quadratic term $\left(r(k+j) - \hat{y}(k+j)\right)^T Q_1 \left(r(k+j) - \hat{y}(k+j)\right)$ and the superscript T denotes the transpose of a vector. The objective function (6.3) is minimized by calculating the future control signals over the control horizon N_u such that the predicted outputs over the prediction horizon N_y are as close to the reference values as possible. Q_1 and Q_2 are weight matrices which relate the relative influence of the deviations of predicted outputs from the corresponding reference values at every future sampling time in the N_y horizon and the control movements in the N_u horizon. The matrices have positive elements and are often chosen as diagonal matrices. The computation of the control signal is based on constraints on both output and manipulated variables:

$$\begin{aligned} y_{min}(k) \leq y(k+j) \leq y_{max}(k) \\ u_{min}(k) \leq u(k+j) \leq u_{max}(k) \\ |\Delta u(k+j)| \leq \Delta u_{max}(k) ... \end{aligned} \tag{6.4}$$

It is also possible to define constraints on the state variables. This can occur when some state variables are allowed to take values only within specific ranges. Also, physical rules can be satisfied with such constraints; for example, a concentration variable cannot be negative, and thus, a minimum zero constraint should be added for the corresponding state.

$$x_{min}(k) \leq x(k+j) \leq x_{max}(k) \tag{6.5}$$

If all state variables are not measured, an observer such as the Kalman filter can be used for estimating these nonmeasurable states. Considering a linear system that can be described by (6.2), Kalman filter can estimate the unmeasurable states vector $x(k)$ as follows:

$$\begin{aligned} K_f(k) &= P_f(k)C^T \left(CP_f(k)C^T + R_f\right)^{-1} \\ x(k+1) &= Fx(k) + Gu(k) + K_f(k)\left(y(k) - Cx(k)\right) \\ P_f(k+1) &= F\left(I - K(k)C\right)P(k)A^T + Q_f \end{aligned} \tag{6.6}$$

where K_f, P_f, R_f and Q_f represent the Kalman gain, error covariance matrix, covariance of measurement, and process noises, respectively.

The standard Kalman filter is an effective tool for estimation, but it is limited to linear systems. Most real-world systems are nonlinear, in which case nonlinear Kalman filters such as extended Kalman filter (Ljung 1979; Knobbe and Buckingham

2005) or unscented Kalman filter (Julier and Uhlmann 2004; Wan and Van Der Merwe 2000; Turksoy et al. 2016, 2017c) is used.

The MPC is formulated with the estimated state variables obtained from the Kalman filter. The block diagram in Fig. 6.1 has an extra observer block which is fed the process input and outputs variables for state estimations. The estimated state variables from the observer are used as the feedback information to the MPC block.

It is also possible to incorporate measured disturbances into calculations of the future behavior of the process outputs for better prediction of the system behavior. Measured disturbances are measurable inputs that are affecting the process behavior but cannot be manipulated by a controller (Fig. 6.1). The state-space model is modified by adding a disturbance term for known (measurable) disturbances $d(k)$ as:

$$\begin{aligned} x(k+1) &= Fx(k) + Gu(k) + Md(k) + v(k) \\ y(k) &= Cx(k) + w(k) \end{aligned} \tag{6.7}$$

The MPC is tuned by adjusting several parameters such as the sampling interval, control and prediction horizons, weight matrices, and filter (observer) parameters by using some guidelines:

- To achieve a good control performance, the sampling interval should be small enough to capture the dynamics of the process and large enough to be able to complete all computations within the sampling interval. Larger sampling intervals may decrease the effect of the control actions on the processes.
- When the control horizon is shorter than the prediction horizon, usually a slower and less aggressive MPC is designed.
- Longer prediction horizons usually result in more forceful control action. The controller becomes more sensitive to disturbances. The stability is influenced by the prediction horizon, and short prediction horizons may cause oscillations in the process outputs.
- The weight matrices are used to adjust the aggressiveness of the control actions. When the control penalty in the objective function is increased, the controller becomes more conservative and yields smoother control actions. However, this may cause slower action in controlled variables to reach the reference values.
- When a deadbeat observer is used, a fast response to disturbances is obtained. The system reacts strongly on high-frequency variations in the process outputs. When disturbances cause frequent saturations in actuators, it is better to tune the observer to be slower to achieve a low filtering effect in the feedback loop.

6.3 Adaptive Control

Generalized Predictive Control

An adaptive controller can modify itself in response to changes in the characteristics and dynamics of the system being controlled (Fig. 6.2). Generalized predictive con-

Fig. 6.2 GPC block diagram

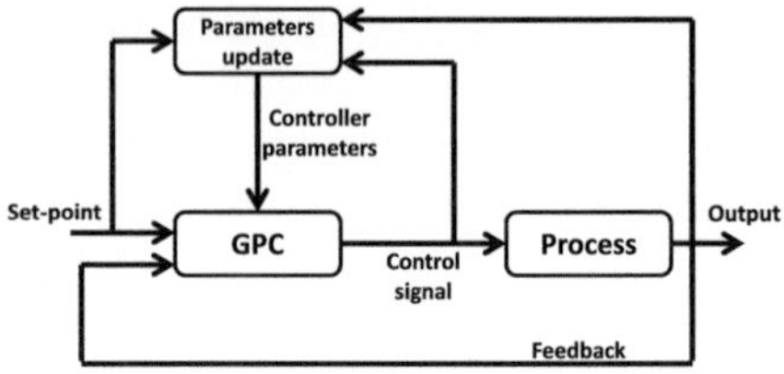

trol (GPC) is a popular adaptive control technique in industry. For time-varying and nonlinear systems, responses to the same disturbances will yield outputs of different magnitudes and characteristics depending on the current state of the system. An adaptive controller uses a frequently updated linear model for regulating such systems. GPC is an adaptive model-based controller (Clarke et al. 1987a, b; Tsang and Clarke 1988; Clarke and Mohtadi 1989). The four components of MPC are valid for GPC as well. GPC is a receding horizon method that depends on predicting the output of a system over several steps into the future based on assumed future control actions and selects the optimal future control moves by minimizing an objective function. The objective function includes terms that represent the deviations of future output trajectories from reference values and penalties about excessive control actions. The fundamental difference from MPC is the model used in GPC algorithm, a low-order linear model updated with every new measurement from the system, thus tracking the changes in system dynamics. The ARMAX model (Chap. 4) in Eq. 6.8 is a general multi-input linear model representation called multivariable ARMAX or vector ARMAX (VARMAX):

$$A(q^{-1})y(k) = q^{-d_i} B_i(q^{-1})u_i(k) + C(q^{-1})e(k) \tag{6.8}$$

where $y(k)$ is the system output, $u_i(k)$ is the ith input variable at kth sampling time, $e(k)$ is the residual at kth sampling time, and d_i is the delay term for the corresponding input. The polynomials A, B, and C are defined as:

$$\begin{aligned} A(q^{-1}) &= 1 + a_1 q^{-1} + a_2 q^{-2} + \cdots + a_{na} q^{-na} \\ B_i(q^{-1}) &= b_{1_i} q^{-1} + b_{2_i} q^{-2} + \cdots + b_{nb_i} q^{-nb_i} \\ C(q^{-1}) &= 1 + c_1 q^{-1} + c_2 q^{-2} + \cdots + c_{nc} q^{-nc} \end{aligned} \tag{6.9}$$

where q^{-1} is the backward shift operator, and n_A, n_{B_i}, n_C are model orders to be determined from data. In GPC algorithm, the ARMAX model is used to predict the system's future outputs. GPC provides the optimal control signal computed by minimizing the quadratic objective function:

$$J(N_1, N_2, N_u) = \sum_{j=N_1}^{N_2} \left[\hat{y}(k+j) - r(k+j)\right]^2 + \sum_{j=1}^{N_u} w(j)\left[\Delta u(k+j-1)\right]^2 \tag{6.10}$$

where N_1 and N_2 are the first and last time instants of the modeling horizon and N_u is the control horizon. $r(k)$ is the reference trajectory, and $w(j)$ is a relative weight for penalizing the control input.

In classical GPC, predicted values are calculated using the Diophantine equation (Clarke et al. 1987a, b; Tsang and Clarke 1988; Clarke and Mohtadi 1989). An alternative is to convert the time series models to state-space models that avoids the computing intensive Diophantine equations (Turksoy et al. 2013a, c).

A significant concern is the possibility of unknowingly developing unstable models at the recursive identification step and using them in the estimation of future output trajectories. This will affect the computation of the optimal control signals. Various methods have been proposed for checking the stability of time series and state space models (Badwe et al. 2010; Lacy and Bernstein 2002, 2003; Lyashevskiy and Chen 1997; Siddiqi et al. 2008). The development of a recursive identification technique that guarantees model stability is more appealing. In this approach, time series models are converted to state-space form. The parameters of the state-space models (originally parameters of the time series models) are found with a constrained numerical optimization. A state-space model is asymptotically stable if all eigenvalues of state matrix are inside a unit circle. The constrained algorithm finds the optimum solution while all eigenvalues of the state-space models are guaranteed to be within the stability region (Turksoy et al. 2013c, 2014b). This numerical solution is equivalent to the analytical solution of the regular RLS method (See Sect. 4.3). Once the model parameters are identified, the model is used for prediction of future values to be used in the objective function (6.10) of the GPC controller. An optimal sequence of future control actions is computed over the control horizon by minimizing the objective function.

Adaptation in MPC Algorithms. Two different approaches have been proposed to provide adaptation in MPC-based AP control. The first approach modifies the objective function based on the values of several parameters (Gondhalekar et al. 2016; Chakrabarty et al. 2017). The MPC law controls BGC to a diurnally time-dependent zone, and enforces diurnal, hard input constraints. The algorithm uses asymmetric input costs in the objective function to improve safety by facilitating the independent design of the MPC responses to hyperglycemia and hypoglycemia. It implements pump suspension in the face of impending (predictive) hypoglycemia. The second approach is inspired by run-to-run control of batch system operation (Palerm et al. 2008; Srinivasan et al. 2001). The parameters of the model used in the MPC are adjusted based on the prediction accuracy of the models and controller performance on the previous day (Palerm et al. 2008; Magni et al. 2009; Toffanin et al. 2017a, b).

6.4 Knowledge-Based Fuzzy Logic Control

Knowledge-based systems (KBS) (also called expert systems) have been used in process industries since 1990s with success. They are based on "If-Then" rules to arrive to a solution based on the conditions satisfied in various rules. Early KBSs were describing facts as well as the rationale to reach conclusions by using rules, which was very inefficient since thousands of rules were generated to describe the current values of measurements. Later, the object- and rule-based hybrid KBS structures were developed. This enabled the use of class–object structures with inheritance to reduce the number of rules drastically and create an efficient reasoning system (Cinar et al. 2007; Tatara and Çinar 2002; Ündey et al. 2003). As the complexity of the system and problem increased, many rules were generated, necessitating a systematic search of rules (depth-first or breadth-first) and prioritizing of the importance of each rule to enable conflict resolution. The next major improvement in KBS technology was the use of fuzzy logic so that the ability to consider more than one possible outcome based on variations in the probabilities assigned to specific outcomes could be incorporated to the KBS. The KBS methodology incorporates a rule-based solution seeking approach to decision-making problems by mimicking various decision-making activities of human beings for making inferences, rather than attempting the development of mathematical models and algorithms. Rules associate ideas and relate the state of some events to initiate or prevent other events. In fuzzy machines, the decision and the means of choosing that decision are based on fuzzy sets and fuzzy rules. A fuzzy set is a set without a crisp, clearly defined boundary. It can contain elements with only a partial degree of membership. This is in contract with deterministic sets that either includes or excludes any given element.

KBS with fuzzy logic has been used in meal detection and meal size estimation (Samadi et al. 2017), detection and discrimination of concurrent MESS factors such as psychological stress during physical activity (Fig. 7.5), and AP control. The fuzzy logic-based AP systems provide a simple way to arrive at a definite conclusion based upon vague, ambiguous, imprecise, noisy, or missing input information by mimicking and automating how a medical expert would make decisions (Fig. 6.3).

The methodology of fuzzy control consists of selecting and using:

- A collection of rules that describe the control strategy,
- Membership functions for the linguistic labels in the rules,
- Logical connectives for fuzzy relations,
- A defuzzification method.

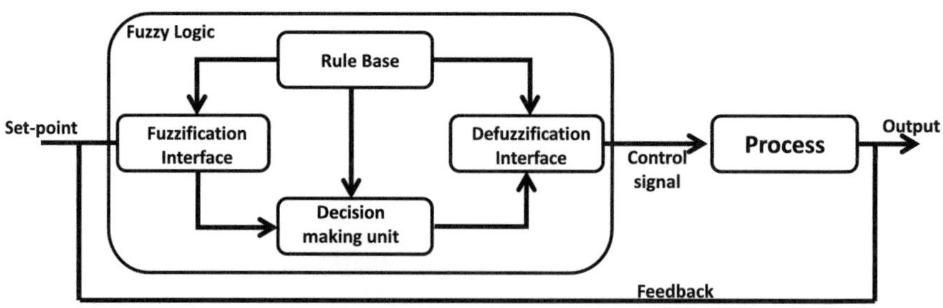

Fig. 6.3 MD-Fuzzy logic block diagram

Various fuzzy logic KBS have been proposed and evaluated in clinical studies for use in APs. Both APs have been developed by collaborative teams that included medical experts and software developers and rely on CGM signals in their control logic. MD-Logic (MD—medical doctor) has been tested in various clinical studies conducted in various countries around the world, and the technology is recently licensed by Medtronic (Atlas et al. 2010; Nimri et al. 2012; Phillip et al. 2013; Nimri et al. 2014a). The Dose Safety FL (FL–fuzzy logic) controller has conducted feasibility studies and stress tests with high carbohydrate/high-fat meals and exercise (Mauseth et al. 2013, 2015).

Chapter 7
Multivariable Control of Glucose Concentration

Abstract The complexity of glucose homeostasis presents a challenge for tight control of blood glucose concentrations (BGC) in response to major disturbances. The nonlinearities and time-varying changes of the BGC dynamics, the occurrence of nonstationary disturbances, time-varying delays on measurements and insulin infusion, and noisy data from sensors provide a challenging system for the AP. In this chapter, a multimodule, multivariate, adaptive AP system is described to deal with several of these challenges simultaneously. Adaptive control systems can tolerate unpredictable changes in a system, and external disturbances by quickly adjusting the controller parameters without any need for knowledge of the initial parameters or conditions of the system. Physiological variables provide additional information that enable feedforward action for measurable disturbances such as exercise. Integration of control algorithms with hypoglycemia alarm module reduces the probability of hypoglycemic events.

Keywords Multivariable artificial pancreas · Biometric variables
Meal detection · Fault detection and diagnosis · Hypoglycemia prediction
Exercise classification

The multivariable control approach leverages real-time information from wearable devices to detect the changes in the metabolic state of a person that can affect BGC. Since the information captured by the biometric (physiological) variables before BGC begins to change, insulin flow rate adjustment can be made sooner to reduce the magnitude of BGC variations caused by MESS and prevent hypoglycemia or hyperglycemia. The multivariable modeling and control framework have:

1. Algorithms for recursive modeling of BGC dynamics by using information from CGM and wearable device(s),
2. Algorithms for interpretation of CGM and wearable device data to determine the presence and the characteristics of MESS,
3. Algorithms and rules to use the data from sensors and the results of data interpretation in item 2 to make alarm and control decisions.

In this chapter, recursive model development for describing glucose concentration variations is introduced (Sect. 7.1), and the use of such models for hypoglycemia

A. Cinar and K. Turksoy, *Advances in Artificial Pancreas Systems*,
SpringerBriefs in Bioengineering, https://doi.org/10.1007/978-3-319-72245-0_7

detection and rescue CHO suggestion is illustrated (Sect. 7.2). Then, the incorporation of algorithms to improve the response of the AP to MESS effects is discussed, focusing on meals (Sect. 7.3), physical activity (Sect. 7.4), acute psychological stress (Sect. 7.5), and sleep (Sect. 7.6). The adaptive controller based on generalized predictive control and the multi-input single-output recursive model of BGC dynamics is introduced in Sect. 7.7.

7.1 Recursive Model of Glucose Concentration Dynamics

Recursive time series models (Sect. 4.3) can describe the time-varying dynamics of BGC by adapting the model with every new measurement. A multi-input single-output ARMAX model is used to describe BGC dynamics, and the ARMAX models can easily be extended to multi-input single-output systems (Sect. 4.2).

$$A(q^{-1})y(k) = B_i(q^{-1})u_i(k-1-d_i) + C(q^{-1})\varepsilon(k) \tag{7.1}$$

where $y(k)$ is the observation (system output) at time k, $u_i(k-1)$ the ith input, $\varepsilon(k)$ white noise, and d_i the delay term for input i. Polynomials A, B, and C are defined in (6.9), and the model orders are determined from data. Writing the ARMAX model in linear regression form (Sects. 4.2.4 and 4.3):

$$\hat{y}(k) = \phi(k)^T\hat{\theta}(k) \tag{7.2}$$

$$\begin{aligned}\phi(k) = [&-y(k-1) \ \cdots \ -y(k-n_A) \quad u_1(k-1-d_1) \\ &\cdots \ u_1\left(k-n_{B_1}-d_1\right) \ \cdots \ u_m(k-1-d_m) \\ &\cdots \ u_m\left(k-n_{B_m}-d_m\right) \quad e(k-1) \ \cdots \ e(k-n_C)]^T\end{aligned} \tag{7.3}$$

$$\begin{aligned}\hat{\theta}(k) = [&a_1 \cdots a_{n_A} \ b_{0_1} \ \cdots b_{n_{B_1}} \\ &\cdots \quad b_{0_m} \cdots b_{nB_m} \ c_1 \ \cdots \ c_{n_C}]^T\end{aligned} \tag{7.4}$$

where $\phi(k)$ and $\hat{\theta}(k)$ are the vectors of past observations and model parameters, respectively, and $e(k)$ is the modeling error that replaces $\varepsilon(k)$ in (7.1):

$$e(k) = y(k) - \hat{y}(k) = y(k) - \phi(k)^T\hat{\theta}(k) \tag{7.5}$$

The optimum coefficients of the ARMAX model are obtained by minimizing the objective function:

$$V\left(\hat{\theta}\right) = \sum_{k=1}^{N} \lambda^{N-k} e(k)^2 \tag{7.6}$$

where N is the number of samples and λ is the forgetting factor.

The model parameters $\hat{\theta}(k)$ (Eq. 7.4) are recomputed (Sect. 4.3) with every new measurement and the resulting model Eq. (7.1) where $e(k)$ is substituted for $\varepsilon(k)$

used until the next measurement. When the disturbance acting on the system is nonstationary, RLS may estimate coefficients that are outside the stability region. A constrained RLS method must be used to guarantee the stability of the models. Furthermore, constraints such as (6.5) are added in the computation of the parameters to have physiologically correct parameter values; for example, insulin can only have a negative effect on BGC. This cannot be ascertained with regular identification methods. For example, if BGC is increasing and insulin is infused at time k, if BGC continues to increase at time $k + 1$, regular identification methods may compute model parameter values that may reflect that the increase is caused by insulin infused at time k. To prevent this erroneous interpretation, all coefficients in Eq. (7.1) related to insulin must be negative to provide the negative effect of insulin on BGC. Otherwise, the model can predict that insulin increases the BGC in some instances. Furthermore, when insulin is administered subcutaneously, diffusion to reach the bloodstream causes a lag and delays glucose utilization. Action curves of subcutaneously administered rapid-acting insulin indicate an estimate action lag of about 15 min, peak action reached in 45–90 min, and the duration of its effect lasting for 3–5 h. The model order of terms related to insulin must be high enough as a function of sampling time to satisfy this physiological fact. Seven different curves were proposed as prediction models of insulin accumulation in the body, also called insulin on board (IOB) (Walsh and Roberts 2006). Regular identification methods may give more weight to older infused insulin than recent ones. To ensure that recently infused insulin has more effect on glucose levels, the coefficients of insulin-related terms in the model must be constrained with minimum values that can be obtained from IOB prediction models. For example, based on the two-hour IOB curve, the coefficients corresponding to $u(k-2)$, $u(k-3)$, and $u(k-4)$ in the ARMAX model can have the minimum values of -0.90, -0.81, and -0.70, respectively.

A stability criterion for the model in Eq. (7.1) can be defined more efficiently in state-space form (Turksoy et al. 2013a). The conversion of the time series model to state space yields:

$$\begin{aligned} \tilde{X}(k) &= \tilde{A}\tilde{X}(k-1) + \tilde{B}\tilde{u}(k-1) + \tilde{K}e(k) \\ y(k) &= \tilde{C}\tilde{X}(k-1) + \tilde{D}\tilde{u}(k-1) + e(k) \end{aligned} \tag{7.7}$$

with

$$\tilde{A} = \begin{bmatrix} -[a_1 \cdots a_{n_A}] & & [b_{1_1} \cdots b_{B_1}] & & \cdots & [b_{1_m} \cdots b_{B_m}] & & [c_1 \cdots c_{n_C}] & \\ I_{p\times p} & 0_{p\times 1} & 0_{p\times r_1} & 0_{p\times 1} & \cdots & 0_{p\times r_m} & 0_{p\times 1} & 0_{p\times s} & 0_{p\times 1} \\ 0_{1\times p} & 0 & 0_{1\times r1} & 0 & \cdots & 0_{1\times r_m} & 0 & 0_{1\times s} & 0 \\ 0_{r_1\times p} & 0_{r_1\times 1} & I_{r_1\times r_1} & 0_{r_1\times 1} & \cdots & 0_{r_1\times r_m} & 0_{r_1\times 1} & 0_{r_1\times s} & 0_{r_1\times 1} \\ \vdots & \vdots & \vdots & \vdots & \cdots & \vdots & \vdots & \vdots & \vdots \\ 0_{1\times p} & 0 & 0_{1\times r1} & 0 & \cdots & 0_{1\times r_m} & 0 & 0_{1\times s} & 0 \\ 0_{r_m\times p} & 0_{r_m\times 1} & 0_{r_m\times r_1} & 0_{r_m\times 1} & \cdots & I_{r_m\times r_m} & 0_{r_m\times 1} & 0_{r_m\times s} & 0_{r_m\times 1} \\ 0_{1\times p} & 0 & 0_{1\times r_1} & 0 & \cdots & 0_{1\times r_m} & 0 & 0_{1\times s} & 0 \\ 0_{s\times p} & 0_{s\times 1} & 0_{s\times r_1} & 0_{s\times 1} & \cdots & 0_{s\times r_m} & 0_{s\times 1} & I_{s\times s} & 0_{s\times 1} \end{bmatrix} \tag{7.8}$$

where $p = n_A - 1$, $r_i = n_{B_i} - 2$ (for $i = 1, \ldots, m$), and $s = n_C - 1$

$$\tilde{D} = \begin{bmatrix} b_{0_1} & \cdots & b_{0_m} \end{bmatrix}, \ \tilde{u}(k-1) = \begin{bmatrix} u_1(k-1-d_1) \\ \vdots \\ u_m(k-1-d_m) \end{bmatrix} \tag{7.9}$$

$$\tilde{C} = \left[-[a_1 \cdots a_{n_A}][b_{1_1} \cdots b_{B_1}] \cdots [b_{1_m} \cdots b_{B_m}][c_1 \cdots c_{n_C}] \right] \tag{7.10}$$

$$\tilde{K} = \begin{bmatrix} 1 & 0 & \cdots & 0 & 0 & 0 & \cdots & 0 & \cdots & 0 & 0 & \cdots & 0 & 1 & 0 & \cdots & 0 \end{bmatrix}^T \tag{7.11}$$

$$\tilde{X}(k-1) = \begin{bmatrix} \begin{bmatrix} y(k-1) \\ y(k-2) \\ \vdots \\ y(k-n_A \end{bmatrix} \\ \begin{bmatrix} u_1(k-1-d_1-1) \\ u_1(k-1-d_1-2) \\ \vdots \\ u_1(k-1-d_1-n_{B_1}) \end{bmatrix} \\ \vdots \\ \begin{bmatrix} u_m(k-1-d_m-1) \\ u_m(k-1-d_m-2) \\ \vdots \\ u_m(k-1-d_m-n_{B_m}) \end{bmatrix} \\ \begin{bmatrix} e(k-1) \\ e(k-2) \\ \vdots \\ e(k-n_C \end{bmatrix} \end{bmatrix}, \ \tilde{B} = \begin{bmatrix} b_{0_1} & \cdots & b_{0_m} \\ 0 & 0_{1\times(m-2)} & 0 \\ \vdots & \vdots & \vdots \\ 0 & 0_{1\times(m-2)} & 0 \\ 1 & 0_{1\times(m-2)} & 0 \\ 0 & 0_{1\times(m-2)} & 0 \\ \vdots & \vdots & \vdots \\ 0 & 0_{1\times(m-2)} & 0 \\ \vdots & \vdots & \vdots \\ 0 & 0_{1\times(m-2)} & 1 \\ 0 & 0_{1\times(m-2)} & 0 \\ \vdots & \vdots & \vdots \\ 0 & 0_{1\times(m-2)} & 0 \\ 0 & 0_{1\times(m-2)} & 0 \\ 0 & 0_{1\times(m-2)} & 0 \\ \vdots & \vdots & \vdots \\ 0 & 0_{1\times(m-2)} & 0 \end{bmatrix} \tag{7.12}$$

The constrained version of the objective function in (7.6) leads to the following minimization problem for computing $\hat{\theta}(k)$ (Turksoy et al. 2013a)

$$\begin{gathered} \hat{\theta}(k) = \underset{\hat{\theta}(k)}{\arg min}[\Delta\theta^T \tilde{P}^{-1}(k-1)\Delta\hat{\theta} + e(k)^2] \\ s.t. \ \rho(\tilde{A}) \leq 1 \\ \hat{\theta}_{min} \leq \hat{\theta}(k) \leq \hat{\theta}_{max} \\ \Delta\hat{\theta} = \hat{\theta}(k) - \hat{\theta}(k-1) \end{gathered} \tag{7.13}$$

where $\tilde{A}$ is the state matrix of the state-space representation of the ARMAX model (7.1) and $\rho(\tilde{A})$ is its spectral radius. The first constraint in (7.13) satisfies the stability condition of the model, and the second one satisfies the physiological properties. $\tilde{P}(k)$

is the estimate of the error covariance matrix (defined in 4.47), and usually $\tilde{P}(0)$ is selected as diagonal matrix.

An adaptive time-varying λ to the weighted recursive least squares (WRLS) algorithm improves performance and data tracking in presence of nonstationary disturbances:

$$\lambda_1(k) = \alpha_1 \lambda(k-1) + (1-\alpha_1)\lambda_0 \tag{7.14}$$

$$\lambda_2(k) = e^{-\left(\frac{e(k-1)^2}{\alpha_2}\right)} \tag{7.15}$$

$$\lambda(k) = \lambda_1(k)\,\lambda_2(k) \tag{7.16}$$

where α_1 is the filter constant that influences how fast λ converges to its final value. Small values of α_1 speed up convergence. λ_0 is the final value of λ when the variance of $e(k)$ (7.5) is small. α_2 is the tuning parameter that adjusts the sensitivity of changes in λ based on the variance of the error. $\lambda(k)$ in (4.47) is updated with every new measurement.

Once the unknown parameters are identified, the predictions of BGC can be obtained at each sampling time by using

$$M = \begin{bmatrix} \tilde{C}\tilde{A}^{N_1-1} \\ \tilde{C}\tilde{A}^{N_1} \\ \tilde{C}\tilde{A}^{N_1+1} \\ \vdots \\ \tilde{C}\tilde{A}^{N_1+N_y} \end{bmatrix} \tag{7.17}$$

$$L = \begin{bmatrix} \tilde{D} & 0 & 0 & \cdots & 0 \\ \tilde{C}\tilde{A}^{N_1-1}\tilde{B} & \tilde{D} & 0 & \cdots & 0 \\ \tilde{C}\tilde{A}^{N_1}\tilde{B} & \tilde{C}\tilde{A}^{N_1-1}\tilde{B} & \tilde{D} & \cdots & 0 \\ \vdots & \vdots & \vdots & \ddots & 0 \\ \tilde{C}\tilde{A}^{N_u-2}\tilde{B} & \tilde{C}\tilde{A}^{N_u-3}\tilde{B} & \tilde{C}\tilde{A}^{N_u-4}\tilde{B} & \cdots & \tilde{D} \\ \vdots & \vdots & \vdots & \cdots & \vdots \\ \tilde{C}\tilde{A}^{N_1+N_y-1}\tilde{B} & \tilde{C}\tilde{A}^{N_1+N_y-2}\tilde{B} & \tilde{C}\tilde{A}^{N_1+N_y-3}\tilde{B} & \cdots & \tilde{C}\tilde{A}^{N_1+N_y-N_u}\tilde{B} \end{bmatrix} \tag{7.18}$$

$$\begin{aligned} \hat{\boldsymbol{y}} &= [\,\hat{y}(k+N_1)\ \hat{y}(k+N_1+1)\ \cdots\ \hat{y}(k+N_1+N_y)\,]^T \\ \tilde{\boldsymbol{u}} &= [\,\tilde{u}(k)\ \tilde{u}(k+1)\ \cdots\ \tilde{u}(k+N_u-1)\,]^T \end{aligned} \tag{7.19}$$

$$\hat{\boldsymbol{y}} = \boldsymbol{L}\tilde{\boldsymbol{u}} + M\left[\left(\tilde{A} - \tilde{K}\tilde{C}\right)\tilde{X}(k-1) + \tilde{K}y(k) + \left(\tilde{B} - \tilde{K}\tilde{D}\right)\tilde{u}(k-1)\right] \tag{7.20}$$

where N_1 and $N_1 + N_y$ are the first and last time instants of the prediction horizon and N_u is the control horizon. $\hat{y}$ is the predicted value of system output (glucose concentration). Note that the first part of the right side of (7.20) depends on future values of manipulated variables. Under an open-loop condition, future values of manipulated variables are unknown and the optimum predictions can be obtained using only the second part of the equation. Integration of the future values of the manipulated variables is shown later in Sect. 7.7.

7.2 Hypoglycemia Detection and Carbohydrate Suggestion

The recursive ARMAX model developed can be used for predicting future BGC values to be utilized in the predictive hypoglycemia early alarm (HEA) system. Figure 7.1 illustrates the working logic of the HEA system which targets 30-minutes-ahead prediction of potential hypoglycemia. Based on measured glucose concentration (CGM) values, five different phases are defined in Fig. 7.1. For

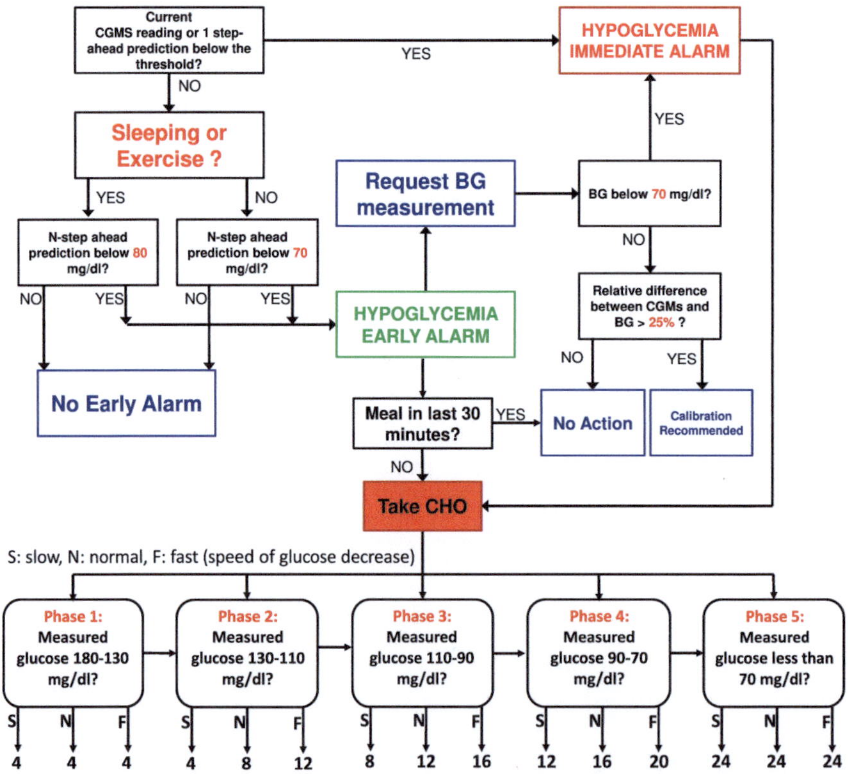

Fig. 7.1 Hypoglycemia detection and carbohydrate suggestion (Turksoy et al. 2018). © 2018 IEEE

each phase, three different speeds of glucose decrease ($\mathring{S}$: slow, $\mathring{N}$: normal, $\mathring{F}$: fast) are defined as

$$speed = \begin{cases} \mathring{S}, & -30 \leq \mathring{\theta} \\ \mathring{N}, & -60 \leq \mathring{\theta} < -30 \\ \mathring{F}, & \mathring{\theta} < -60 \end{cases} \tag{7.21}$$

$$\mathring{\theta} = \tan^{-1}\left[\frac{\sum_{i=k-N_{CHO}}^{k}\left(\mathring{x}_{i-k+N_{CHO}} - \mathring{X}\right)(y_i - Y)}{\sum_{i=0}^{N_{CHO}}\left(\mathring{x}_i - \mathring{X}\right)^2}\right] \tag{7.22}$$

where $\mathring{x} = [0, 5, 10, 15, 20, 25]$ (based on 5 min sampling time) and y_k is measured glucose at time k. $\mathring{X}$ and Y are mean values of $\mathring{x}$ and y_i $(i = k - N, \ldots, k)$, respectively. The moving window length N_{CHO} is selected to be 5 (last 30 min). With every new measurement, 30-minutes-ahead glucose predictions are compared with the 70 mg/dl mild hypoglycemia threshold (80 mg/dl during exercise). If the predicted values are below the threshold, the last measured glucose value is used for determination of the phase interval. At the same time, the speed of glucose reduction is obtained using (7.21) and (7.22). Once the phase and the speed of reduction are calculated, specific amounts of CHO (Fig. 7.1) are suggested to patients for consumption. Only one CHO consumption suggestion is done in one phase (except phase 5) until glucose levels decrease to the next level.

7.3 Meal Detection and Hyperglycemia Prevention

The meal detection algorithm is based on detection of rapid increases in glucose concentration in the absence of a specific reason besides meal consumption. Other conditions may be sensor error, which does not need any insulin bolus or other physiological reasons that may sharply reduce insulin sensitivity, which may need insulin boluses. Sensor errors are treated by fault detection and diagnosis algorithms. Two different meal detection and insulin bolus calculation algorithms are outlined below to illustrate the use of two different paradigms. The first algorithm is based on using a compartmental physiological model and estimating some unmeasured variables by a Kalman filter for detecting the presence of a meal. The second algorithm relies on qualitative trend description of CGM profiles over time and use of fuzzy logic to detect a meal. Both algorithms also provide suggestions for insulin boluses to be infused. The algorithms are tuned to be aggressive in identifying meals but conservative in bolus insulin dose administration to prevent the potential for hypoglycemia due to overdose of insulin.

Meal Detection with a Physiological Model. A compartmental model is used to detect the effects of a meal. The first three-compartment "minimal model" to analyze plasma glucose and insulin dynamics during an intravenous glucose tolerance test was developed in Bergman et al. (1981). The dynamical equations for plasma glucose concentration $G(t)$ and effective insulin concentration I_{eff} are given by Roy and Parker (2006)

$$\frac{dG(t)}{dt} = -p_1 G(t) - p_4 I_{eff}(t) G(t) + p_1 G_b + R_a(t) \tag{7.23}$$

$$\frac{dI_{eff}(t)}{dt} = -p_2 I_{eff}(t) + p_3 I_p(t) \tag{7.24}$$

where G_b and I_p represent basal plasma glucose concentration and plasma insulin concentration, respectively. The rate of appearance of glucose $R_a(t)$ can be defined as a two-compartment model (Hovorka et al. 2004)

$$R_a(t) = \frac{C(t)}{V\tau^2} t e^{-\frac{t}{\tau}} \tag{7.25}$$

where $C(t)$, V, and τ are the amount of consumed CHO, the distribution volume, and the peak time of meal absorption, respectively. In the original "minimal model" in Bergman et al. (1981) and its extensions in (Hovorka et al. 2002; Roy and Parker 2006) the unknown model parameters p_1, p_2, p_3, p_4, V, and τ are not time-varying. However, due to the complexity of the human body and intra-subject variability, a constant set of parameters may not be able to describe all time-varying dynamics for a subject. Also, inter-subject variability may require different sets of parameters for different subjects. In this method, all unknown parameters and the basal BGC G_b are defined to be time-varying in order to accommodate the inter- and intra-subject variability. Using the first forward difference derivative approximation, (7.23)–(7.25) are discretized and G_b is defined as

$$G_b(k) = \begin{cases} 100, & k < \frac{2l}{h} \\ \frac{h}{l}\sum_{i=k-\frac{2l}{h}+1}^{k-\frac{l}{h}} G_s(i), & k \geq \frac{2l}{h} \end{cases} \tag{7.26}$$

where h represents sampling time and l is the length of the window that is used for calculation of G_b and selected to be 30 min.

A meal detection algorithm based on estimation of the unmeasurable variables in (7.23)–(7.25) is developed. The real-time estimations are obtained using unscented Kalman filter (Julier and Uhlmann 2004; Wan and Van Der Merwe 2000; Turksoy et al. 2016, 2017c). When the estimated $R_a(k)$ values are above the threshold of $2\,[mg/dl/min]$, a meal bolus is considered to be infused. If BGC keeps increasing in spite of the infused insulin (meal) bolus, a series of mini-correction boluses are suggested. The correction boluses are calculated based on measured CGM values $G_s(k)$ and a subject's body weight (BW) as a function of total daily dose (TDD) as follows

$$CB = \frac{G_s(k) - y_{ref}(k)}{1800} \times TDD \tag{7.27}$$

TDD can be approximately estimated from the *BW* and insulin sensitivity constant (ISC) of a patient

$$TDD = ISC(k) \times BW \tag{7.28}$$

Insulin sensitivity is subject-specific and time-varying. Thus, a time-varying *ISC* is defined as a function of glucose predictions in (7.20) and reference trajectory

$$ISC\,(k) = \hat{y}\,(k)\,./y_{ref}\,(k) \tag{7.29}$$

where ./ indicates element-wise division. The reference trajectory vector y_{ref} is defined iteratively

$$y_{ref}\,(k+j) = \mu y_{ref}\,(k+j-1) + (1-\mu)y_{ref_0} \tag{7.30}$$

where y_{ref_0} is the constant "set point" and indicates the desired value of the trajectory. $y_{ref}(k)$ is set equal to $y(k)$ at the first iteration ($j = 1$). The parameter $\mu \in [0, 1]$ determines the speed of approximation of the reference trajectory to y_{ref_0} such that the closer μ is to 1, the smoother is the approximation.

Meal Detection with Fuzzy Logic. Meal detection and meal size estimation can also be based on qualitative description of segments of CGM values over time represented by triangular shapes (Fig. 7.2), followed by fuzzy logic decision making to determine the start time of the meal and its amount (Samadi et al. 2017). After a meal is identified, a fuzzy system estimates the amount of CHOs consumed during the time window labeled as the meal consumption period. The meal size estimator uses both CGM and insulin data. The meal insulin bolus is based on the total estimated CHOs in the meal.

The algorithm uses three different techniques, wavelet filtering, qualitative representation analysis, and fuzzy logic, to detect meals and estimate their amounts. A wavelet filter is used to reduce the CGM signal noise level. Qualitative representation of the filtered CGM signal assigns one of the seven qualitative variables to each episode, and the signs of the first and second derivatives within an episode are determined. This information is used in the rules that determine the presence of a meal and its CHO amount. Frequent information from the CGM is crucial for early detection of changes in the state of the system. At every sampling time, a new

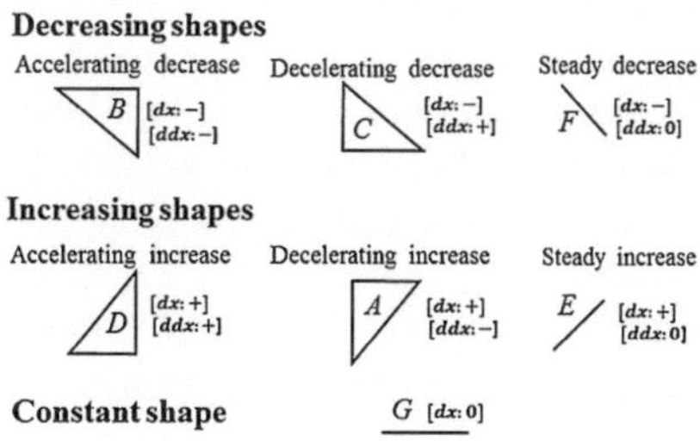

Fig. 7.2 Seven shapes assigned to different types of CGM change trends over time (Samadi et al. 2017). © 2017 IEEE

episode is considered. All episodes have the same length, and two adjacent episodes may take the same qualitative variable. The amount of CHO consumed is estimated as the meal continues during the meal consumption period and mini-boluses can be infused according to CHO amounts estimated at successive sampling times.

To date, only a few studies have investigated the detection of meals from real-time measurable variables such as CGM measurements. Some of these studies address only meal detection, while some others propose methods for meal size estimation as well as meal bolus suggestions with meal detection. A voting algorithm based on Kalman filter estimation, backward difference, combination of Kalman filter and backward difference, and second derivative of CGM measurements was proposed in Dassau et al. (2008). A meal is considered to be detected when two-out-of-three or three-out-of-four algorithms detects a meal. A meal detection and meal size estimation algorithm was developed in Lee et al. (2009). The algorithm was combined with model predictive control-based AP system. Meal times and sizes are estimated based on various thresholds and if/then rules using first and second derivatives of glucose measurements. A probabilistic method for meal detection was developed in Cameron et al. (2009). First, CGM signals are compared to no-meal predictions made by a simple insulin–glucose model. The residuals are fitted to predefined meal shapes used for detection of meals. Later, the method was extended for use in a model predictive control algorithm for blood glucose regulation (Cameron et al. 2012a). A variable state dimension-based method was developed in Xie and Wang (2017). The method identifies two data-driven state-space glucose concentration models (the number of states is different in two models) with and without meal as one of the input. Meals are detected by a Kalman filter that switches its operation between the two models. Meal sizes are estimated using some predefined statistics (Xie and Wang 2017).

7.4 Physical Activity

Physical activity provides a major challenge to AP systems, because the effect, magnitude, and physiology of this perturbation is not well understood, and real-time information about the characteristics of a physical activity on the body are not considered in the algorithms of the AP. The effects of physical activity vary from person to person, and with the type, intensity, and duration of the activity. Physical activity could be unplanned (running to catch a bus), unstructured (house cleaning, group sports), or structured (daily exercise routines). Several studies and publications on physical activity, especially structured exercise, have been presented in Sect. 3.2. It is known that mild- and medium-intensity physical activities usually induce hypoglycemia in T1D due to increased glucose uptake as well as inadequate glucagon secretion and/or hepatic glucagon sensitivity. However, different types of exercise, such as aerobic or resistance exercise, as well as the duration and intensity of this exercise, have different effects on the incidence of hypoglycemia. The lack of physiological models of insulin action and glucose uptake during exercise prevents quantification of the effect of exercise on insulin sensitivity as well as other variables, especially in T1D. Another complication arises because alcohol consumption can also cause hypoglycemia, but by a different mechanism, so an AP system needs to be sophisticated enough to recognize the difference by using other physiological inputs and take corrective action accordingly.

The multivariable AP approach addressed exercise detection and mitigation of its effects by a two-prong approach (Turksoy et al. 2013b, 2014a). A multi-input model was developed to include physiological information from data collected from a sports armband (Andre et al. 2006) in order to improve the accuracy of BGC prediction. Recursive identification was used to update the model when new data were collected to adapt the model continuously to the present state of the person. In addition, the physiological information (energy expenditure and galvanic skin response) was used to indicate automatically the beginning and end of an exercise period, to be additional inputs to the recursive model, and to incorporate rules to the control logic such that the insulin infusion rate computed is adjusted automatically in presence of exercise. The clinical experiments indicate the success of the multivariable AP in regulating BGC in spite of various unannounced meals and exercises as indicated in Fig. 7.3.

Exercise Classification. The identification of the type and intensity of exercise and its reliance on aerobic or anaerobic metabolism provide useful information to the control logic of the AP since their effects on BGC are different. The type of exercise (aerobic versus resistance/anaerobic) can be determined by a k-nearest neighbors (KNN) classification algorithm (Turksoy et al. 2015). KNN classification does not formulate a generalized conceptual model from the training instances at the training stage. Rather, a simple and intuitive rule is used to make decisions at the classification stage: Instances close in the input space are likely to belong to the same class. An

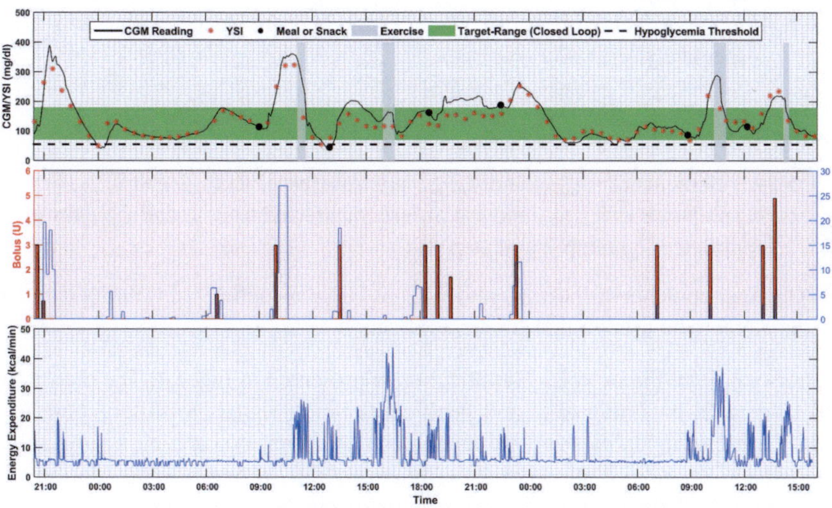

Fig. 7.3 Performance of the Multivariable AP in a clinical experiment

object is classified by a majority vote of its neighbors, with the object being assigned to the class most common among its k-nearest neighbors.

Defining $\breve{x}$ and $\breve{y}$ as the matrix of input features and vector of output labels of a training dataset, the standardized Euclidean distance vector $D_{\breve{x},\breve{x}_{new}}$ between a new observation vector $\breve{x}_{new}$ and training data matrix $\breve{x}$ is defined as

$$D_{\breve{x},\breve{x}_{new}}(t) = \sqrt{\sum_{j=1}^{\breve{m}} \left(\frac{\breve{x}_j(t) - \breve{x}_{new,j}}{W_j} \right)^2} \tag{7.31}$$

where $t = 1, \ldots, \breve{N}$ and $\breve{N}$ is the number of training data and W_j is the standard deviation of jth column of $\breve{x}$ matrix for N observations. The KNN algorithm is:

1. Compute the distance $D_{\breve{x},\breve{x}_{new}}(t)$ for all $t = 1, \ldots, \breve{N}$.
2. Select k lowest distance and corresponding $\breve{y}(t)$.
3. Select $\breve{y}_{new}$ as the most frequent class from the previous step.

If there are outliers in training data, the KNN algorithm may have some incorrect classification, similar to all other data-based classification algorithms. Condensed nearest neighbors (CNN) rule (Hart 1968) was proposed to decrease the size of training data to a minimum such that the reduced size data are still able to describe all training data. The CNN algorithm is:

1. The first sample $\breve{x}(1)$ and $\breve{y}(1)$ is placed in $\breve{x}_{store}$ and $\breve{y}_{store}$, respectively.
2. The second sample $\breve{x}(2)$ is classified by the KNN algorithm using $\breve{x}_{store}$ and $\breve{y}_{store}$
   a. If $\breve{x}(2)$ is classified correctly, $\breve{x}(2)$ and $\breve{y}(2)$ are placed in $\breve{x}_{discard}$ and $\breve{y}_{discard}$, respectively.
   b. If $\breve{x}(2)$ is not classified correctly, $\breve{x}(2)$ and $\breve{y}(2)$ are placed in $\breve{x}_{store}$ and $\breve{y}_{store}$, respectively.
3. Repeat step-2 for all $\breve{N}$ ($t = 1, \ldots, \breve{N}$) observation in training data.
4. Use $\breve{x}_{discard}$ and $\breve{y}_{discard}$ and repeat step 2 and step 3 until:
   a. All elements of $\breve{x}_{discard}$ and $\breve{y}_{discard}$ are transferred to $\breve{x}_{store}$ and $\breve{y}_{store}$, or
   b. No elements of $\breve{x}_{discard}$ and $\breve{y}_{discard}$ are transferred to $\breve{x}_{store}$ and $\breve{y}_{store}$ during a complete loop (step-2 and step-3).
5. The final contents of the $\breve{x}_{store}$ and $\breve{y}_{store}$ are used as optimized training data for the KNN to be used in real-time classification.

An example of the exercise classification is presented in Fig. 7.4. The algorithm uses heart rate, breathing rate, and peak acceleration signals to differentiate and classify exercise modalities and the reliance on an exercise on aerobic or anaerobic metabolism. The algorithm classifies erroneously only a few readings during the switching times between aerobic and anaerobic activity due to complexity in data during these transients changes from one mode of exercise to another (Turksoy et al. 2015).

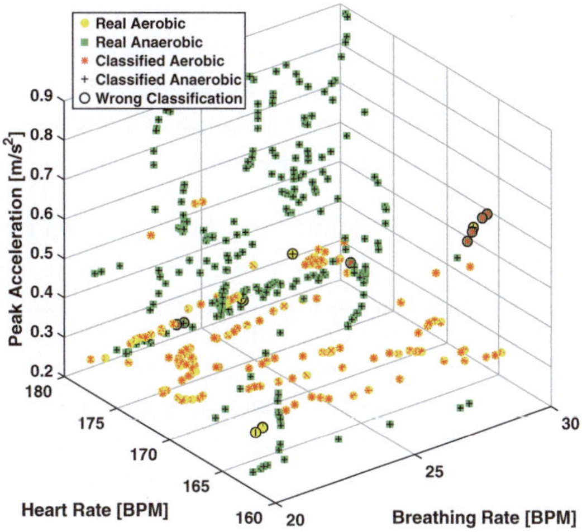

Fig. 7.4 Classification of aerobic and anaerobic (resistance) exercise in real time. Wrong classifications occurred mostly during transitions between the two types of exercise (Turksoy et al. 2018). © 2018 IEEE

Various studies investigated the effects of including biometric variables in AP systems to improve performance and mitigate exercise-induced hypoglycemia. This is a precursor to a multivariable approach, akin providing meal information. Information about the beginning and end of a known type of exercise was generated and used, but the variables that indicated physical activity were not incorporated in the predictive models to develop multi-input models and the control decisions were often limited to insulin suspension. A method to detect the start and end of exercise in people with T1D before any significant change in BGC occurred was proposed by collecting outpatient ambulatory data from accelerometer (ACCM), heart rate (HR), CGM, insulin pump, and glucose meter for the first two days of the study to inform the detection algorithm (Dasanayake et al. 2015). On the third day, subjects performed aerobic exercise for 1 h at 30% predicted maximal heart rate reserve in the morning and for 30 min at 50% heart rate reserve in the afternoon. Subjects were then discharged and collected data for two more days. Principal component analysis was used for activity detection due to the high correlation between heart rate and acceleration data. The study concluded that this detection method identified the onset and end of exercise in approximately 5 min, with an average BG change of −6 mg/dL.

Free-living data from subjects with T1D were collected using a combined ACCM and HR, an insulin pump, and a CGM in order to supplement an existing predictive low glucose suspend algorithm (Stenerson et al. 2014b). The different algorithms were tested in a computer simulation and compared based on reduction in exercise-related hypoglycemia. The low glucose suspend algorithm reduced hypoglycemia by 62%, while the HR-augmented algorithm and the ACCM-augmented algorithm reduced hypoglycemia by 71% and 74%, respectively. Combined HRM and ACCM use reduced hypoglycemia by 76%. In a follow-up study (Stenerson et al. 2014a), the effectiveness of the ACCM-augmented low glucose suspend algorithm was compared with the subjects regular basal insulin rate during an outpatient exercise protocol.

An on-algorithm soccer session and an off-algorithm soccer session where the rate of hypoglycemia during and after exercise was compared. The difference in meter glucose levels between groups did not achieve statistical significance at any time, and the ACCM-augmented algorithm failed to prevent hypoglycemia compared to subjects on their usual basal rates.

The performance of a control-to-range (CTR) AP with a CTR system informed by heart rate (CTR+HR) was compared based on the following metrics: BGC decline during exercise, the low BGC index (LBGI), number of hypoglycemic episodes (BGC < 70 mg/dl), and overall glucose control (% time with BGC between 70 and 180 mg/dl) (Breton et al. 2014). Twelve subjects participated in two 26 h sessions including 30 min of mild exercise. The CTR+HR system significantly reduced BG decline during exercise, marginally reduced LBGI, allowed fewer hypoglycemic events during exercise, and increased the time within the target BGC range. LBGI and average BG remained constant. Despite small sample size, the study achieved statistically significant results showing that BGC rate of decline during exercise was reduced when HR information was supplied to the closed-loop controller. However, this study was only a special case where subjects had no cardiovascular complications and performed only mild exercise, and the HR signal collection was triggered manually rather than starting based on automated detection of exercise.

In another study, CGM and heart rate variability (HRV) data were gathered from ten subjects with T1D while bedridden during insulin-induced hypoglycemia. These data were used to develop an algorithm to detect hypoglycemic periods based on pattern recognition to decide whether the BGC would be below 3.9 mmol/L at a certain point in time. For a ten-minute prediction, the algorithm provided 79% sensitivity (true positive hypoglycemia rate) and 99% specificity (true negative hypoglycemia rate), detecting 16/16 hypoglycemic events with no false positives and a 22-minute lead time compared to the CGM alone (Cichosz et al. 2014). In a follow-up study, the researchers used this pattern classification algorithm to predict hypoglycemia based on three different models: (i) a model containing raw CGM data; (ii) a model containing data derived from CGM signal; and (iii) a model containing data derived from CGM and HRV signals. Twenty-one subjects were monitored while performing normal daily activities to predict spontaneous hypoglycemia. For a 20-minute-ahead prediction, model (i) resulted in a ROC AUC of 0.69 and had a 69% specificity for a 100% sensitivity, model (ii) had a ROC AUC of 0.92 with a 71% specificity for a 100% sensitivity, and model (iii) had a ROC AUC of 0.96 with a 91% specificity for a 100% sensitivity. Combining CGM and HRV data improved hypoglycemic prediction (Cichosz et al. 2014).

7.5 Acute Psychological Stress

Acute stress causes rapid increase in BGC. This must be differentiated from BGC increases caused by meals. Physiological variables from wearable devices can provide this distinction and also inform the AP about the stress before the rise in BGC.

Most variables measured by wearable devices available in the market are affected both by stress and physical activity. For example, heart rate and galvanic skin response (GSR) respond to both stimuli. Hence, several variables need to be considered for differentiating the presence of stress versus physical activity. Accelerometer information can provide this distinction for some types of exercise, since the individual may not necessarily move in many stress situations. But the challenges increase as one considers the variaties of exercise types. For Example, many wearables do not detect riding a bicycle when a wristband is worn since the person's arms are not moving. A GPS signal can detect bicycling on the road, but not stationary bicycling. The determination of exercise and stress becomes even more challenging when both are present at the same time. This is a common situation in sports competitions.

The information reported by wearable sensors must be interpreted to detect the presence of one or more MESS factors, then discriminate whether the reported values indicate a meal, exercise, stress or sleep, or a combination of them. The AP can formulate the proper course of action to mitigate their effects only after the correct diagnosis and classification are made. The ability to detect and discriminate various MESS factors necessitates careful selection of physiological variables to measure. For example, accelerometers, heart rate, and GSR would change for both aerobic and anaerobic exercise. Additional variables or analysis in the patterns of measured variables will be necessary to discriminate between various types and intensities of exercise (Turksoy et al. 2015). Both the selection of physiological variables that carry the necessary information and the interpretation of their values are critical for the success of multivariable AP systems to mitigate the effects of MESS. The contributions of powerful data interpretation algorithms that work on the feature space may be necessary. Some techniques that have been successful in these cases have been discussed, and the discrimination of competition stress, social stress, and no stress states by using data from wearable devices with good accuracy have been reported (Sevil et al. 2017). The availability of information about acute stress in real time will improve decision making about insulin infusion rates by considering the variation in insulin sensitivity.

Progress has also been made in detecting and discriminating the presence of concurrent acute psychological stress during physical activity. The patterns of a derived signal indicate when a subject is exercising without or with mental stress, or having mental stress or not during a sedentary state (Fig. 7.5).

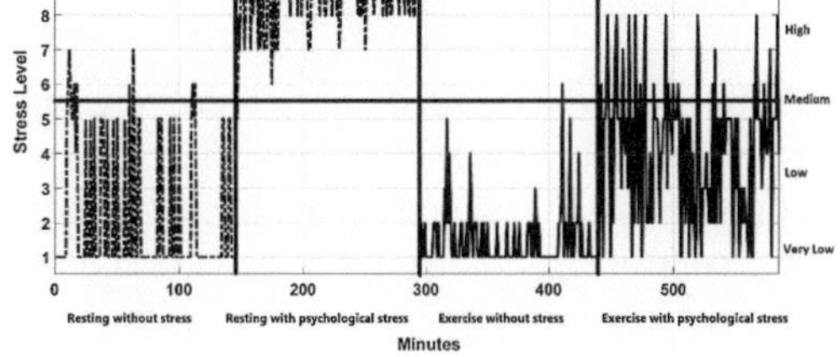

Fig. 7.5 Detection and discrimination of acute psychological stress (mental stress) during sedentary state and medium-intensity exercise

7.6 Sleep

Almost half of hypoglycemic events occur during the overnight periods while sleeping due to unawareness of low glucose levels (DCCT Research Group and Others 1991). Consequently, automatic control algorithms for AP systems that can accommodate the effects of sleep are in obtaining euglycemia during night. Such control algorithms need more information than what glucose concentrations can provide. Any individual variable such as heart rate, accelerometer, posture, or galvanic skin response can provide information to indicate and discriminate sleep. Once the sleep condition is detected, AP settings or hypoglycemia thresholds can be adjusted accordingly (Turksoy et al. 2013c, b).

Several sleep-specific problems have been addressed with AP technology. Many clinical studies with closed-loop control at night have been reported with glycemic control results better than multiple daily insulin injections and sensor-augmented pump use (Thabit et al. 2015; Bally et al. 2017; Brown et al. 2015; Renard et al. 2016; Kropff et al. 2015; Russell et al. 2016; Nimri et al. 2014b; Kumareswaran et al. 2011). Hypoglycemia detection has been integrated into many AP systems to modify insulin infusion rates as needed. Some systems such as the Medtronic MiniMed 630 G rely on the current CGM reading for determining hypoglycemia, in line with the first step of the original JDRF road map (Sherr et al. 2014). Many researchers developed algorithms based on BGC predictions to make inferences about potential hypoglycemia and adjust insulin infusion rates 25–30 min in advance of a potential hypoglycemia episode (Turksoy et al. 2014a, 2013c; Buckingham et al. 2010; Beck et al. 2014; Buckingham et al. 2015). Commercial systems available outside of the US have also adopted the predictive hypoglycemia approach (Medtronic MiniMed 640 G).

A glucose sensor problem during sleep, PISA, has also been addressed. PISA is caused by pressure on the region where the CGM is located when body position changed during sleep, causing variations in CGM readings that are not related to BGC variations. Various algorithms have been developed to detect and mitigate the effects of PISA (Baysal et al. 2014; Feng et al. 2017; Turksoy et al. 2017b). AP control strategies that tighten control in early morning hours to bring BGC in range by the time the person with T1D wakes up have been proposed (Forlenza et al. 2017). Preliminary results indicate that this improves BGC control during the following day.

7.7 Multivariable Adaptive Control

Various model-based predictive control algorithms propose different cost functions for obtaining the control law (Sect. 6.3). The general aim is that the future output $\hat{\boldsymbol{y}}$ on the horizon considered should follow a reference signal $\boldsymbol{y}_{ref}$, while the magnitude of the control effort $\boldsymbol{u}$ should be penalized as shown in (6.10).

The constrained control signal is calculated by minimizing

$$\tilde{\boldsymbol{u}}_1(k) = \arg\min_{\tilde{u}_1} \left[\left(\hat{y} - y_{ref}\right)^T (\hat{y} - y_{ref}) + \Delta\tilde{\boldsymbol{u}}_1{}^T w \Delta\tilde{\boldsymbol{u}}_1) \right] \\ s.t.\ \tilde{\boldsymbol{u}}_{1min} \leq \tilde{\boldsymbol{u}}_1 \leq \tilde{\boldsymbol{U}}_{1max} \tag{7.32}$$

where only the first element of $\tilde{\boldsymbol{u}}_1(k)$ is implemented. Since the model in (7.1) is created as a multi-input model, $\tilde{\boldsymbol{u}}_1$ represents the first column (defined to be insulin) of $\tilde{\boldsymbol{u}}$ that is the future value matrix of all inputs. The AP system uses insulin as the only manipulated variable. Any external input variables in (7.1) that are not manipulated by the controller are fed to the objective function in (7.32) externally. The external inputs are modeled with separate autoregressive moving average (ARMA) models for prediction of future values to be used in (7.32)

$$A_i(q^{-1})\tilde{u}_i(k) = C_i(q^{-1})\varepsilon_i(k) \tag{7.33}$$

$$\tilde{\boldsymbol{u}}_i = M_i \left[\left(\tilde{A}_i - \tilde{K}_i\tilde{C}_i \right) \tilde{X}_i\,(k-1) + \tilde{K}_i\tilde{u}_i(k) \right] \text{ for } i = 2, \ldots, m \tag{7.34}$$

where M_i, $\tilde{A}_i$, $\tilde{K}_i$, $\tilde{C}_i$, and $\tilde{X}_i(k-1)$ are calculated by following from (7.2) to (7.17).

One of the challenges in closed-loop control of BGC is the lack of information about how much BGC decreases with one unit of insulin for a specific patient, also known as the insulin sensitivity factor (ISF). The more sensitive a patient is to insulin, the greater the glucose decline for each unit of insulin administered. The 1500 and 1800 rules are generally used for calculating ISF without any clinical measurements (Hanas and Ragnar Hanas 2009). These rules are suitable for most patients with T1D. However, like many properties of BGC dynamics, ISF is also subject-specific and time-varying. Additional rules have been proposed for generalization (Walsh et al. 2010). ISF can be used for calculating $\tilde{\boldsymbol{u}}_{1max}$ in (7.32). It can be expressed as a function of the TDD

$$ISF = 1800/TDD \tag{7.35}$$

The amount of insulin accumulated in the body (for details, see "Rapid-Acting Insulin Analogs") can be predicted as

$$IOB\,(k+j) = IOB_{crv}[\,\tilde{u}_1(k-1+j)\ \cdots\ \tilde{u}_1(k-n_{B_1}+j)\,]^T \tag{7.36}$$

where IOB_{crv} is a column vector with elements in the range [0, 1] obtained from one of the 7 insulin-on-board (IOB) curves (Walsh and Roberts 2006) and $j = 1, 2, \cdots, N_u$. The $\tilde{\boldsymbol{u}}_{1max}$ in (7.32) is defined as

$$\tilde{\boldsymbol{u}}_{1max}\,(k+j-1) = \left(\frac{\hat{y}\,(k+j) - y_{ref}\,(k+j)}{ISF} \right) - IOB(k+j) \tag{7.37}$$

The weight matrix w in (7.32) is assigned values by relating it to ISF update for each subject adaptively

$$w = diag(ISF) \tag{7.38}$$

An alternate to these equations based on generalized values is the use of plasma insulin concentration estimates. Estimators based on the extensions of Hovorka's model have been proposed by making some of the model parameters additional state variables (Hajizadeh et al. 2017; de Pereda et al. 2016).

Adaptation in the multivariable framework has been implemented by using the GPC approach (Sect. 6.3) and recursive models of glucose concentration dynamics (Sect. 7.1) and utilizing additional modules for hypoglycemia, meals, exercise, fault detection and data reconciliation, and controller performance assessment retuning. Additional modules for mitigating the challenges caused by stress and sleep and for fault-tolerant control would improve the performance of the multivariable adaptive AP.

Chapter 8
Dual-Hormone (Insulin and Glucagon) AP Systems

Abstract AP systems that use both insulin and glucagon to regulate BCG can provide control that mimics the performance of the pancreas more realistically. The added complexity of control algorithms and hardware, the current stage of development of long-term stable glucagons provide challenges to the dual-hormone AP system. The progress made by various research groups is reported.

Keywords Glucagon · Stability · Dual hormone artificial pancreas

Most AP systems are single-hormone systems that achieve closed-loop glycemic control by administering insulin in response to changing physiological conditions detected by CGM and other sensors. However, the slow onset and prolonged effect of insulin analogs when delivered subcutaneously means that until a more rapidly acting insulin preparation is available, suspension of subcutaneous insulin during impending hypoglycemia may be insufficient to prevent hypoglycemia (Castle et al. 2010; El-Khatib et al. 2014). Dual-hormone AP systems endeavor to mimic the biological pancreas more realistically and address this issue by administering both insulin and glucagon in response to changes in BGC. In dual-hormone AP systems, glucagon is given as mini-boluses to prevent or treat hypoglycemia while insulin infusion is suspended (Taleb et al. 2017).

Several studies were published by one group (The Boston Group) since 2010 investigating the dual-hormone AP systems in pigs and humans (El-Khatib et al. 2010). The first human study took place in a controlled, sedentary environment with standardized meals. The AP was reactive, using an MPC to determine subcutaneous insulin dosing and a PID with an online accumulation term to determine subcutaneous glucagon dosing. Glucagon was absorbed more rapidly than insulin lispro, allowing for a rapid positive change in the time derivative of BGC to prevent postprandial hypoglycemia. However, this rapid onset of glucagon action does not help prevent hypoglycemia if too much excess insulin was allowed to accumulate due to sustained differences between model glucose values and measured glucose val-

A. Cinar and K. Turksoy, *Advances in Artificial Pancreas Systems*,
SpringerBriefs in Bioengineering, https://doi.org/10.1007/978-3-319-72245-0_8

ues (El-Khatib et al. 2010). In a study reported in 2012, a meal-priming bolus was added to the system, and CGM measurements were used instead of venous BGC measurements. This system was automated except for meal-priming boluses, and it automatically adapted to a subject's needs in real time. The system achieved good BGC control with minimal hypoglycemia. However, it struggled to regulate postprandial hyperglycemic excursions encountered by every AP due to the absorption delay of subcutaneously infused insulin and the delay in CGM measurements relative to BGC variations. The CGM underestimated BGC during hyperglycemia and in some instances failed to detect hypoglycemia indicated by BGC measurements. There were also technical issues involving pump failure (Russell et al. 2012). The researchers reported a third-generation AP in inpatient and outpatient environments, designed to respond to glycemic changes on multiple time scales to account for both short-term and long-term changes in insulin requirements within and between individuals while being initialized only with the subjects weight (El-Khatib et al. 2014). Results show that this AP can adapt in less than 24 h to safely and effectively regulate glycemia in adolescent and adult populations with T1D and with highly variable insulin requirements. Adolescents required more time for the AP to adapt to achieve effective insulin dosing due to higher insulin requirements and lower body mass, resulting in higher mean BGC and requiring adaptive meal-priming boluses (El-Khatib et al. 2014). In the outpatient study with this AP, the researchers compared glycemic control with a wearable version of this AP and glycemic control by using an insulin pump for five days in 20 adults and 32 adolescents with T1D. The system used an automatically adaptive algorithm whose only inputs were CGM data and estimates of meal size to control subcutaneous delivery of insulin and glucagon. The results of this study showed that the AP improved mean glycemic levels and allowed fewer hypoglycemic episodes to occur in adults and adolescents (Russell et al. 2014).

In another dual-hormone AP, insulin and glucagon administration were adjusted according to a fading memory proportional derivative (FMPD) algorithm. In this algorithm, recent errors were weighted more heavily than earlier errors, and the difference between the current glucose level and the target level as well as the rate of change of glucose were used to adjust insulin and glucagon administration. Glucagon was given to some subjects using high-gain parameters and to other subjects using low-gain parameters only if hypoglycemia was imminent. The system was not fully closed-loop because subjects received a meal-priming bolus after a meal announcement. Despite mean glucose levels being similar between the high-gain glucagon and placebo studies, the subjects who received automated high-gain pulses of glucagon along with insulin delivery experienced fewer hypoglycemic events, spent less time in the hypoglycemic range, and required fewer treatments with oral CHOs compared to subjects who received a placebo along with insulin (Castle et al. 2010). In 2014, the "Oregon group" reported an inpatient study with a second-generation AP. In addition to the FMPD controller with meal announcement used previously, a physiologic model of insulin and glucose metabolism was included to estimate each subjects varying insulin sensitivity in order to modify the gains of the PD controller. In both APs, glucagon administration was not required; glucagon was only delivered for rescue purposes. Results from these and other closed-loop clinical trials have demonstrated that closed-loop control can lead to glucose levels in the euglycemic range of 70–180 mg/dL approximately 70% of the time (Jacobs et al. 2014).

In a third dual-hormone AP, real-time CGM readings were entered to a computer that calculated insulin and glucagon delivery. Insulin and glucagon were given manually through infusion pumps. Meal announcement with CHO counting was required to calculate prandial boluses (Haidar et al. 2013). Each experiment included exercise on a stationary bicycle, one meal, one snack, and an overnight stay. The results showed that dual-hormone closed-loop delivery reduced inter-patient variability in BGC, increased time spent in the target glucose range, and decreased time spent in hypoglycemia compared with insulin pump therapy. There was no increased risk of hyperglycemia. Although mean plasma glucose did not differ between the two treatments, hypoglycemia was common during control visits using insulin pump therapy, so the mean glucose level during those sessions was reduced, while closed-loop delivery eliminated most hypoglycemia without increasing mean glucose levels (Haidar et al. 2013). In 2016, the "Montreal group" reported another study comparing their dual-hormone system with a single-hormone system during announced continuous and interval exercise on an ergocycle in a controlled inpatient environment. For the dual-hormone system, insulin delivery was calculated using an MPC algorithm, while glucagon delivery was calculated using logical rules based on estimates of BGC and its trends. The addition of glucagon to the AP resulted in fewer episodes of exercise-induced hypoglycemia as well as more time spent in the normal glycemic range for both continuous and interval exercise. The amounts of insulin delivered by the two systems were comparable, which suggests that the improvement in glycemic control by the dual-hormone system is attributed only to the addition of glucagon (Taleb et al. 2016).

Another closed-loop dual-hormone AP included a self-learning individualized PD control algorithm to calculate insulin dosing based on proportional error, derivative error, insulin sensitivity, and two glucose thresholds triggering insulin bolus delivery (Van Bon et al. 2012). Glucagon was administered if glucose fell below a threshold. The size of the bolus was dependent on the rate of fall of BGC, and subsequent delivery occurred according to an exponential glucagon injection curve. Glucagon was given in a rescue bolus if hypoglycemia occurred. No meal or exercise announcements were given. The study protocol included two meals and treadmill exercise. Closed-loop control was comparable to open-loop control, but patients with higher baseline glucose received excess insulin. There were no differences in time spent in euglycemia, hypoglycemia, or hyperglycemia or in post-exercise glucose concentrations between open-loop and closed-loop, but more hypoglycemic episodes occurred during closed-loop. Subcutaneous glucagon administration was almost always effective to prevent hypoglycemia when glucose was falling rapidly after exercise (Van Bon et al. 2012). The "Netherlands group" published results from another study investigating the safety and performance of their dual-hormone system compared to insulin pump therapy during short-term daily use in an outpatient environment (Blauw et al. 2016). The same control algorithm was used except that glucagon doses were reduced. The insulin sensitivity factor was initially set based on the subjects weight, but it was reevaluated every day and changed manually if necessary. The dual-hormone system provided better glucose control than insulin pump therapy, most significantly overnight. During the overnight period, more time was spent in euglycemia, less time was spent in hyperglycemia, and the median glucose level was lower for the AP compared to insulin pump therapy. There was no significant difference between the two groups in time spent in hypoglycemia or in the number of CHO-treated hypoglycemic events, which demonstrates that the AP was at least as safe as insulin pump therapy (Blauw et al. 2016).

The dual-hormone AP system is expected to improve glucose control during situations with an increased risk of hypoglycemia, such as exercise, but there are several challenges that still need to be overcome before they become commercially available (Taleb et al. 2016). One major issue is that the approved clinical use of glucagon has been limited to emergency treatment of severe hypoglycemia with a single large bolus (Taleb et al. 2017). Depletion of liver glycogen can occur if too much glucagon is administered. Excessive glucagon delivery can lead to hyperglycemia and nausea (Jacobs et al. 2014). Most pharmacological studies investigating the effects of glucagon have used doses greater than the usual emergency bolus of one milligram, while mini-boluses used in the AP system are usually only on the scale of micrograms. Human studies using these small but relatively frequent glucagon doses are lacking, so long-term AP trials should address questions about the benefits and potential risks of continued glucagon use (Taleb et al. 2017). The lack of an FDA-approved, stable, soluble form of glucagon is another challenge (Peyser et al. 2014). Current formulations of glucagon are stable for only short periods of time due to their tendency to aggregate, which can affect their activity and cause pump occlusion. In order for glucagon to be a reliable addition to an AP system, it would need to be stable and not require reconstitution or replacement for two to three days (Russell 2015).

There is a risk of insulin and glucagon working against each other, causing more insulin to be administered (Russell 2015). Longer human trials of chronic glucagon administration in dual-hormone APs should measure insulin and glucagon sensitivity and resistance, glucose flux, and glycogen stores (Taleb et al. 2017). Also, failure of glucagon delivery would increase the risk of hypoglycemia. However, this risk could be reduced with appropriate tuning of the control algorithm (Russell 2015) and algorithms to detect failures of glucagon delivery. For systems that use model-assisted control, an empirical or physiological model of glucagon action in T1D needs to be developed (Bakhtiani et al. 2013).

T1D is characterized by lack of insulin as well as inappropriately high levels of glucagon secretion and deficient glucagon counter-regulation. Excessive glucagon secretion contributes to ketoacidosis in poorly controlled T1D, and deficient glucagon counter-regulation contributes to hypoglycemia (McCall and Farhy 2013). Although there are challenges associated with the dual-hormone AP, there are compelling reasons to continue working to mitigate these challenges for improving glycemic control in T1D. Even if insulin is dosed correctly, delayed absorption of subcutaneously administered insulin means that the dosing may not be correct by the time it reaches the bloodstream, especially in the case when exercise begins within that time delay. Single-hormone systems can suspend insulin delivery and issue an alarm, but delayed absorption means that suspension may not be sufficient to prevent hypoglycemia, and the alarm may not be effective if the patient cannot respond to mitigate hypoglycemia. Automatic glucagon delivery in a dual-hormone system requires no action from the patient, and glucagon is absorbed more quickly than insulin in subcutaneous delivery (Russell 2015). Up to 60% of hypoglycemic events go unrecognized because they are asymptomatic. Patients with hypoglycemic unawareness might benefit the most from this technology, and larger and longer studies in outpatient setting are needed (Haidar et al. 2013). Dual-hormone APs increase system complexity, potential for system failures, and equipment cost, but glucagon use reduces hypoglycemia risk compared to single-hormone systems (Taleb et al. 2017).

Chapter 9
Fault Detection and Data Reconciliation

Abstract The performance of an AP system depends on successful operation of its components. Faults in sensors other hardware and software affect the performance and may force the system to manual operation. Many AP systems use model predictive controllers that rely on models to predict BGC and to calculate the optimal insulin infusion rate. Their performance depends on the accuracy of the models and data used for predictions. Sensor errors and missing signals will cause calculation of erroneous insulin infusion rates. Techniques for fault detection and diagnosis and reconciliation of erroneous data with reliable estimates are presented. Since the models used in the controller may become less accurate with changes in the operating conditions, controller performance assessment is also conducted to evaluate the performance and determine if it can be improved by adjusting the model, parameters or constraints of the controller.

Keywords Fault detection and diagnosis · Data reconciliation
Controller performance assessment

Reliable operation of an AP depends on the performance of (i) the sensors providing accurate information at a high frequency (sampling time of 5 min for the CGM, 1/60th of a second for some wearable physiological sensors), (ii) the controller that calculates the insulin infusion rate based on sensor signals, (iii) the insulin pump and the interfaces between the body and the sensors and pump, and (iv) the communications between devices. Sensor faults such as signal bias, outliers, pressure-induced sensor attenuation (PISA), and missing data will affect insulin infusion rate calculation and predictive alarms for hypoglycemia and hyperglycemia, endangering the proper operation of the AP and patient safety (Baysal et al. 2014; Del Favero et al. 2014; Facchinetti et al. 2016; Feng et al. 2016b; Turksoy et al. 2017e). Controller performance deterioration affects the insulin infusion rates computed (Feng et al. 2016a). It can be caused by changes in glucose and insulin concentration dynamics of the user and inaccuracies in information received from various sensors and insulin pump. The system (body) and model mismatch increases as the dynamics of the user's metabolism changes over time and causes BGC estimates with poor accuracy unless the model is adapted. Malfunctions in the pump and insulin delivery system and occlusions in the body at the insulin delivery site cause mismatch between the

A. Cinar and K. Turksoy, *Advances in Artificial Pancreas Systems*,
SpringerBriefs in Bioengineering, https://doi.org/10.1007/978-3-319-72245-0_9

intended amount of insulin to be infused and the insulin reaching the bloodstream. Interruptions in communications can cause missing sensor data and outliers that can affect the insulin dose computed. Early work on patient safety focused on detecting hazardous situations from CGM readings and taking appropriate measures (Patek et al. 2012). Recent CGM sensors and pumps also have error-checking capabilities as part of their firmware. Techniques in fault detection and diagnosis, and in data reconciliation provide faster detection of abnormalities in the operation of the AP and reliable estimates for missing or erroneous sensor readings. This chapter focuses on sensor error detection, reconciliation of data to provide more "realistic" information from the sensors to the control system, and the assessment of controller performance and the modification of the controller over time.

9.1 Sensor Error Detection and Data Reconciliation

Fault detection algorithms can be grouped into three categories: qualitative model-based methods, quantitative model-based methods, and process history-based (data-driven) methods (Venkatasubramanian et al. 2003). The process history-based methods rely on the availability of large amounts of historical process data capturing system behavior under various conditions. Relations between variables, patterns that indicate various abnormalities, statistical limits that indicate significant deviations are extracted from the historical data and used for fault detection. Their performance depends on the richness of information and quality of historical data. Model-based fault detection methods can be developed by using compartmental models based on first principles such as material and energy balances. Qualitative model-based methods use knowledge-based (expert) systems and may not be appropriate by themselves for fault detection in complex biological systems. A knowledge-based system uses if-then-else rules that mimics the reasoning of a human expert in solving problems. As the number of if-then-else rules grows with the behavioral complexity of the system, some rules may conflict with the new rules and the maintenance of the system and conflict resolution may become challenging (Cinar et al. 2007).

Kalman filter, Extended Kalman Filter (EKF) (Facchinetti et al. 2011; Baysal et al. 2014), support vector machines (Bondia et al. 2008; Leal et al. 2013a), wavelets (Shen et al. 2010; Campetelli et al. 2011), kernel-density-based stochastic model (Signal et al. 2012), rates-of-change-threshold-based model (Baysal et al. 2013) and principal components analysis (PCA) (Leal et al. 2013b; Cinar et al. 2007; Turksoy et al. 2017b, e) methods have been used for detection of CGM failures. Detection of pressure-induced sensor attenuation (PISA) based on the rate of change in CGM readings was proposed and PISA was defined to be a negatively biased reading (Baysal et al. 2014). A Kalman filter-based method for detecting sudden spikes and loss of sensitivity in CGM was reported where the loss of sensitivity was defined to be negatively biased signals as well (Facchinetti et al. 2013). A kernel-based stochastic modeling technique was used for detection of CGM spikes in data collected from critically ill patients (Signal et al. 2012). A discrete wavelet-transform-based online

CGM dropouts detector was developed (Shen et al. 2010). A method that compared different statistical monitoring charts was reported for detecting unexpected changes in CGM readings (Zhao and Fu 2015). Various studies focused on assessing the correctness of CGM sensor readings rather than detection of sensor failures (Bondia et al. 2008; Leal et al. 2013a, b). EKF is used for state estimation of nonlinear systems (Kandepu et al. 2008); however, the linear approximation at operating point approach in EKF may cause errors when a time-varying model is used. Also, the computation of Jacobian matrices may be challenging with high-order models. The UKF (Julier and Uhlmann 2004) overcomes the drawbacks of EKF and can easily be implemented to high-order systems without calculation of Jacobian matrices.

Two different approaches will be outlined for sensor error detection and reconciliation of information for use by the controller. One approach is based on the use of a compartmental (first principles) model and estimation of changes in some model parameters to infer the presence of sensor errors and reconcile data. The second approach relies on the development of data-driven empirical models by using multivariate techniques to achieve the same objectives. The development of a error detection data reconciliation module that integrates both approaches will also be illustrated to improve error detection accuracy and the performance of functional sensor redundancy for better estimates to replace erroneous data.

A method that combines of model- and process history-based algorithms for detection of CGM-related faults is presented in (Turksoy et al. 2017e). The model-based component is based on an extended Bergman's model. The effects of free fatty acid (FFA) (Roy and Parker 2006) and exercise (Roy and Parker 2007) are included in recent extensions of the MM. Some state variables of the first-principles models (Bergman et al. 1981; Cobelli et al. 1986, 1999; Hovorka et al. 2002; Roy and Parker 2006, 2007) are not measurable. These non-measurable states and model parameters are estimated from available measurements (Kanderian et al. 2009). The time-invariant model parameters of the MM are not appropriate for sensor fault detection because of intra- and inter-subject variability over time. Therefore, model states and parameters are estimated simultaneously by defining uncertain model parameters as augmented states. An unscented Kalman filter (UKF) (Julier and Uhlmann 2004; Wan and Van Der Merwe 2000) is implemented for state estimation. The data-driven portion of the fault detection method is based on principal components analysis (PCA). PCA involves the orthogonal decomposition of the set of process measurements along the directions that explain the maximum variation in the data (Cinar et al. 2007). PCA is used to develop a model that describes the expected variation under normal conditions. Deviations from normal (expected) operation of the sensors is detected if either of the two statistics exceed their limits: the *Hotelling's* T^2 that detects the deviation of a new observation from the reference model and the *squared prediction error SPE* (also called Q charts) that indicate deviations from reference data that are not captured by the PCA model (Cinar et al. 2007).

The T^2 and *SPE* may exceed their limits not only when there is a faulty CGM reading, but also when some dynamic changes not captured in the reference dataset used in model development and computation of T^2 and *SPE* limits. These dynamic changes should not be declared as fault. In order to minimize the number of erroneous fault detections, a two-step fault diagnosis algorithm is developed to distinguish CGM faults from regular dynamic changes (Turksoy et al. 2017e).

After the presence of a fault is detected by either the T^2 or SPE statistics, its source must be determined. This can be achieved by identifying the variables responsible for inflating T^2 and SPE statistics. The variables that made the largest contributions to these statistics are considered to indicate the equipment faults such as specific sensors. Another approach is to develop a list of patterns of specific faults and match the pattern of the current faults to one of the patterns in the list to identify the source cause (Cinar et al. 2007).

A data-driven approach was proposed by using the framework of batch process operation where the length of a batch run is set as one day (24 h) (Turksoy et al. 2017b). The behavior of the body and glucose dynamics in response to daily events that are repeated can be considered as the operation of a batch process. These events include meals and exercise. Glucose levels increase after a meal and they are reduced when insulin is infused. This pattern is repeated for every meal. Exercise causes variation patterns in glucose levels by affecting the sensitivity to insulin and insulin-independent glucose uptake. These sequences of events are repeated during a day and over time.

Several disturbances to glucose homeostasis may occur during different times of a day. Meals cause sharp rises in BGC that taper off slowly to a steady value. Meal times and compositions vary. Physical activity and stress may also occur during at different times from one batch to another. Mismatch in events and event times may cause erroneous interpretations, and it is necessary to align batches to be used for developing the reference that describes the normal operation of the body. Dynamic time warping (DTW), a pattern-matching scheme that works with pairs of patterns to locally translate, compress, and expand the patterns so that similar features in the patterns are matched (Berndt and Clifford 1994) is extended to align trajectories for developing a better reference trajectory. DTW nonlinearly warps two trajectories such that similar events are aligned and a minimum distance between them is obtained. DTW is a pairwise algorithm that requires a reference trajectory to be used for synchronization other trajectories. DTW may suggest aligning one single point on one trajectory to many points of the other trajectory the peaks or valleys in trajectories might be slightly lower (or higher) from one trajectory to another. Use of the point first-order derivative (d^1) instead of Euclidian distance has been suggested as a measure of the difference between two trajectories to overcome this singularity problem (Keogh and Pazzani 2001). Since the datasets considered may not follow a Normal distribution, higher-order moments are also included in the proposed method. This high-order DDTW captures more statistical information by using higher-order derivatives.

The method simultaneously monitors several measurements and detects unexpected readings in real time. The information about unexpected changes or detected faults can be used by the AP to prevent undesirable events and modifying the controller to become more conservative in presence of faults. The proposed algorithm is able to successfully detect various unexpected simultaneous changes in multiple sensors and diagnose their source and nature according to predefined rules.

An alternative data-driven approach integrated sensor fault detection and data reconciliation by using functional redundancy. It uses two types of model that treat data differently. The outlier-robust Kalman filter (ORKF) is a data-driven model in traditional Kalman filter structure that has been used in sensor outlier-related problems in various fields such as global positioning system (GPS) data analysis (Agamennoni et al. 2011) and robotic systems (Ting et al. 2007). Sensor data can be described by Kalman filter equations with hidden states. As a data-driven model for predicting measured values, the data used to train the model has to be robust to outliers. The coefficient matrices representing the system dynamics need to be adaptive to fit dynamic changes in a system with time-varying coefficients. The standard Kalman filter with constant coefficients that considers all data samples to be part of the data cloud would not be appropriate and could generate erroneous estimates. To overcome these limitations, a Bayesian algorithm that treats the weights associated with each data sample probabilistically is introduced. A scalar gamma-distributed weight is assigned for each observed data sample. Gamma distribution is chosen to ensure that they remain positive. The resulting prior distributions are Normal. This entire problem can be treated as an Expectation-Minimization-like (EM) learning problem (Dempster et al. 1977; Ghahramani and Beal 2000) and model parameters can be found by maximizing a log-likelihood function. A forgetting factor is introduced to the ORKF to give more weight to recent data to generate the model, which enables the model to adapt to variations in a system with time-varying parameters (Feng et al. 2017).

The second data-driven model relies on locally weighted regression (LWR) (Cleveland 1979), which constructs a local model by prioritizing samples in a database according to the similarity between them and a query sample. There are many sample sets paired with their prediction values in the database. The locally weighted partial least squares (LW-PLS) compares the current sample with samples in the database and gives a weight for each sample in the database according to their similarity with the query sample and uses the weighed samples to generate a PLS model to predict the query sample (Feng et al. 2017). Comparing a query sample in LW-PLS with all the samples in the database is time-consuming, and not necessary. Clusters enabling the distinction of the basic characteristic (shape) of the samples and comparing the query sample only with the samples that have the same basic characteristic improves diagnosis efficiency. A clustering algorithm generates five different groups (increase period, decrease period, increase followed by decrease period, decrease followed by increase period, and steady period). Historical data clusters are used to develop the PLS models and the confidence limits to determine current data that may indicate abnormalities such as sensor errors (Feng et al. 2017).

The ORKF (Ting et al. 2007) and the LW-PLS (Kim et al. 2013) provide two complementary technologies. ORKF provides predictions of sensor readings based on the recent behavior of the sensor. LW-PLS uses a model developed by historical data and updates its parameters with current sensor information. Consequently, its predictions take into account the historical information about the expected system performance. The two techniques are also used to implement functional redundancy by estimating the likely sensor readings rather than the missing or erroneous data reported. Again, pooling the estimates based on both techniques provides a better estimate rather than using either one of the techniques for data reconciliation (Feng et al. 2017).

False positive error detections, missing errors, and the erroneous signal estimates due to the model inaccuracies are important challenges for SED&FR systems. This occurs more frequently when the dynamic changes in the system are too large or too rapid, and the model used in SED&FR system does not have enough prior information to adapt to such large dynamic changes. Since the criterion for error detection is based on the residual between the measurement and model prediction, large number of false positives can occur. A simple threshold for signal change is not reliable to distinguish between sensor errors and correct sensor readings caused by rapid changes in sensor readings, since rapid dynamic changes can also cause large residuals. The nominal angle analysis (NAA) concept is proposed to distinguish between sensor errors and real dynamic changes in sensor readings and added to the SED&FR system (Feng et al. 2017).

9.2 Controller Performance Assessment and Retuning

A multi-level supervision and modification (ML-SCM) module is developed to supervise the performance of the AP system and modify it to adapt to the patients current metabolic state and mitigate the impact of CGM sensor faults. The ML-SCM module contains three sub-modules based on different timescales: sample-level supervision module (SLSM), period-level supervision module (PLSM), and 24 h day level supervision module (DLSM). An index-based online controller performance assessment (CPA) module (Feng et al. 2016a) and a hybrid CGM sensor error detection and functional reconciliation (SED&FR) module (Feng et al. 2016b) based on outlier-robust Kalman filter (ORKF), and local weighted partial least squares (LW-PLS) were developed for a GPC-based AP (Turksoy et al. 2014b, 2016). These two modules were capable of retuning the controller and reconcile the CGM signal values at each sampling time. In the ML-SCM module, the performance of the AP will not only be assessed at the sample level but also at period level and day level. The CPA module is enhanced with additional indexes to track different aspects of controller performance and combined with SED&FR module to formulate the SLSM (Feng et al. 2018). The dynamic changes in the body triggered by meal or physical activity will last for many sampling times. Hence, the ML-SCM module should accommodate the effects of different situations over various time periods. The PLSM based on linear quadratic Gaussian (LQG) control-based trade-off curve and DLSM based on daily BG distribution analysis are developed to assess the AP performance in longer time scales.

The SLSM has two sub-modules, a CPA and a SED&FR. In previous work (Feng et al. 2016a), an online CPA module with six indexes to track different aspects of a model-based controller such as MPC of GPC was developed. The indexes used in the previous CPA module included model prediction error index, model error elimination speed index, dangerous change potential index, dangerous change index, insulin constraints limitation index, and weight ratio index. Three different types of controller failures, model prediction error, insulin constraints error, and controller objective function weight ratio error, are detected and the controller is modified accordingly. Two additional indexes: idle index (Hägglund 1999) and performance watchdog (Rhinehart 1995) are added to the CPA sub-module to detect sluggish control and offset from set point (reference trajectory), respectively (Feng et al. 2018).

By extending SLSM with PLSM and DLSM, the performance of the controller is improved because PLSM assists in returning the controller for different disturbances such as meals and exercise, and DLSM caused improvements from day to day, akin to run-to-run batch process improvement. DLSM modifies the adjustable range of the parameters in the AP and constraints for insulin boluses.

Chapter 10
Clinical AP Studies

Abstract Clinical studies ranging from investigational experiments to clinical trials that compare alternate treatments and control techniques are listed.

Keywords Clinical studies · AP clinical trials · Outcomes

Ninety-six clinical trials were conducted between 2006 and 2016. The MPC, PID, fuzzy logic, and GPC are used in 61 (Turksoy et al. 2017a) (references 40–100 therein), 25 (Turksoy et al. 2017a) (references 33, 44, 51, 61, 63, 97, 99, 101–118 therein), 8 (Turksoy et al. 2017a) (references 33, 44, 51, 61, 63, 97, 99, 101–118 therein), and 2 (Turksoy et al. 2017a) (references 1, 127 therein) of the experiments, respectively. Overall, 1473 subjects participated in these trials. The first clinical trial, in Austria, was reported in 2006 (Turksoy et al. 2017a) (references 41 therein). Later, many more studies were performed between 2008 and 2016 in the USA (50), UK (17), Italy (9), Israel (9), France (8), the Netherlands (7), Germany (5), Canada (5), Austria (3), Spain (2), Denmark (1), and Slovenia (1) (Fig. 10.1).

Most of the experiments were performed based on subcutaneous glucose measurement and subcutaneous insulin infusion. Some studies used glucagon as the second control action to prevent hypoglycemia (Turksoy et al. 2017a) (references 44, 51,55, 77, 81, 85, 96, 99, 100, 105, 106, 108, 114, 118, 128 therein). Although glucagon works well to prevent low glucose concentration, in almost all reported studies, on some occasions, administration of glucagon alone was insufficient to fully prevent hypoglycemia and additional rescue CHOs were needed.

The most challenging times for the APs tested were postprandial meal periods, when hyperglycemia is seen if an appropriate amount of insulin is not infused in time. Current rapid-acting insulins have nonphysiologic action profiles and are much slower than the insulin produced by the body. Any delays in infusion adds additional delays and may cause hyperglycemia. Even with various proposed meal detection algorithms, an AP system cannot autonomously take action until the effect of meals begins to impact measured glucose concentrations. This is not ideal as it has been

A. Cinar and K. Turksoy, *Advances in Artificial Pancreas Systems*,
SpringerBriefs in Bioengineering, https://doi.org/10.1007/978-3-319-72245-0_10

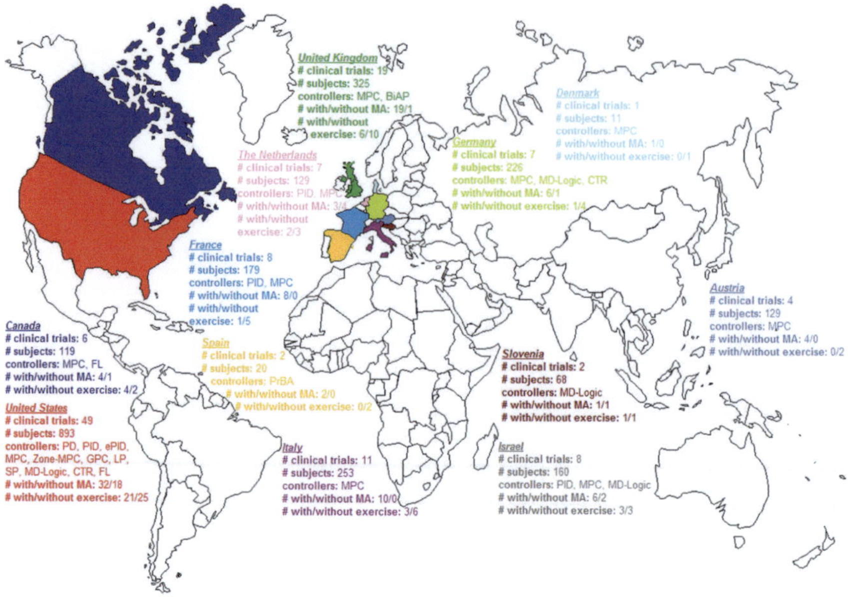

Fig. 10.1 Clinical trials conducted between 2006–2016

found that administering insulin 20 min before the beginning of a meal reduces postprandial hyperglycemia (Turksoy et al. 2017a). To overcome that challenge, most AP systems were developed as hybrid systems where patients still need to enter meal or a bolus insulin dose information into the APs by using their insulin to CHO ratio before the meal. To be fully automated, some studies have tested a no meal announcement approach (Turksoy et al. 2017a) (references 1, 43, 44, 55, 58, 65, 75, 96, 98, 106, 108–111, 114, 118, 119, 123, 124, 127 therein)

Some of these studies used meal detection algorithms that detected meal consumption without any manual announcements (Turksoy et al. 2017a) (references 138–142 therein). If proven viable and successful in larger trials, they can be used in AP systems with no meal announcement to minimize postprandial hyperglycemia (Turksoy et al. 2017a) (references 138–142 therein) and to assist patients who may not compute meal information correctly or forget to enter their meal information.

Physical activity has significant effects on BGC, and it is important that AP systems overcome this hurdle, particularly for children who have many spontaneous physical activities. The first experiments that included exercise sessions were performed in 2010 (Turksoy et al. 2017a) (references 45 therein). Since then, several additional studies incorporating exercise into AP systems have been conducted to study their effects on BGC (Turksoy et al. 2017a) (references 1, 50, 51, 53–55, 60, 61, 75, 81, 84, 88, 93, 95, 99, 100, 108, 113, 120, 123, 126–128 therein). One group used heart rate signals to detect exercise (Turksoy et al. 2017a) (references 60 therein), while another group focused on a multivariable AP that used physical activity signals such as energy expenditure, galvanic skin response, and heart rate from an activity monitor in addition to CGM measurements to better estimate glucose values and to use these signals in the control logic to decrease insulin infusion rates and, if necessary, recommend CHO consumption to prevent exercise-induced hypoglycemia (Turksoy et al. 2017a) (references 1, 127 therein).

The use of AP systems had initially been restricted to the inpatient research setting because of the complexities of such systems. Recent advances and results from AP studies have transitioned AP technology to the outpatient setting. To achieve APs full potential in the outpatient milieu, portable devices such as smartphones and tablets have been employed. A study was undertaken in the inpatient setting to test the feasibility of a smartphone-based AP system for this purpose (Turksoy et al. 2017a) (references 143 therein). The first tests of the APs in an outpatient setting were made in a diabetes camp setting (Turksoy et al. 2017a) (references 40, 63, 123 therein). The first camp study occurred during 2011–2012 and was a multicenter, randomized crossover trial that assessed short-term safety and efficacy of AP for nocturnal glucose levels in subjects 10–18 years old in Israel, Slovenia, and Germany (Turksoy et al. 2017a) (references 123 therein). The first published study of day and night bi-hormonal (insulin and glucagon) control included two 5-day outpatient trials: one testing a bionic pancreas in adults, and another testing the same system in adolescents in a summer camp; both trials had no restrictions on diet or exercise (Turksoy et al. 2017a) (references 63 therein). The first published outpatient insulin-only day and night study tested the AP for 7 days in adults who were advised against vigorous physical activity, but their diet was not restricted (Turksoy et al. 2017a) (references 40 therein). Additional camp studies have been completed recently, in which patients participated in various physical activities (Turksoy et al. 2017a) (references 76, 91, 95, 99, 116, 117 therein). Further outpatient studies have been published, 6 in a hotel or university setting (Turksoy et al. 2017a) (references 33, 57, 64, 75, 83, 86, 87 therein) and 8 in the patients homes (Turksoy et al. 2017a) (references 40, 74, 82, 89, 90, 92, 96, 98, 114, 118, 121, 125 therein). Of the studies conducted at home, only two tested closed-loop control for 24 h a day while the remaining used traditional insulin pump therapy during the day (Turksoy et al. 2017a) (references 64, 90 therein). More technical and detailed information for all completed studies is available in Turksoy et al. (2017a).

Chapter 11
Future Developments

Abstract Various possible future directions in the development of AP systems are discussed. Further development of faster and more stable hormones will make the AP systems to react as fast as the human body. More accurate glucose and wearable sensors with faster response times will enhance the ability of AP systems for better glucose regulation. Integration of biometric variables into AP system will reduce manual information needed from users. A hybrid AP system with manual meal entries is already available. Several companies and research teams are developing more advanced AP systems that are being tested in clinical trials and are expected to become commercially available in the near future.

Keywords Future of artificial pancreas · New technologies and designs

Progress in AP research and development is occurring in many fronts: new hormone formulations, new glucose sensors, wearable devices that provide additional signals to the AP, advanced control algorithms, controller performance assessment and adaptation, fault-tolerant-control and algorithms to predict and mitigate various disturbances. Contributions are made by academic research groups, industry, and individuals.

Research in new hormone formulations are progressing both in ultra-fast-acting insulin development that will improve the speed of impact and clearance of insulin, and in long-term stable glucagon that will enable the development of dual-hormone APs—a system that operates more closely to the way a biological pancreas functions. These developments are complemented by improved pharmacokinetics/pharmacodynamics, and possibly new routes of insulin delivery such as intraperitoneal, intradermal routes.

Developments in glucose sensor technologies are progressing on several fronts. New generations of subcutaneous CGM sensors have better amperometric technologies and fluorescence-based elements to improve measurement accuracy and longer use. These sensors also have improved their data processing algorithms to reduce measurement errors. Developments in fully implantable sensors with longer use peri-

A. Cinar and K. Turksoy, *Advances in Artificial Pancreas Systems*,
SpringerBriefs in Bioengineering, https://doi.org/10.1007/978-3-319-72245-0_11

ods and innovel sensors that measure additional hormones are promising. The latter will enable multivariable AP systems. Another appealing development in sensor technologies is factory-calibrated systems that eliminate capillary BGC measurement with finger sticks for sensor calibration at least every 12 h.

The explosion in wearable device technologies provides the potential to harvest valuable information in real time for MESS disturbances. Devices that provide streaming accurate data since real-time control decisions will be based on the information provided. Measured variables may not be enough to provide the information about the presence, characteristics, and coexistence of MESS events, and feature extraction and interpretation by various data-driven machine learning algorithms must be used to extract knowledge from wearable device data. These data and refined information will also contribute to research on the effects of psychological stress, high-intensity exercise, sleep, illness, and seasonal effects such as menstrual cycles. Some examples of modules that complement the basic AP control system have been discussed in earlier chapters.

Such additional information will also improve fault detection and mitigation, by creating the opportunity to use functional redundancy to estimate missing or erroneous data. One of the goals of the next-generation APs is to provide fault-tolerant AP systems. These APs should be able to mitigate the effects of interruptions in data transmission (sensor data and commands to the pump), equipment failures (sensors, pump, interfaces between devices and the body), and software errors. This should be complemented by controller performance assessment and retuning. The first prototypes of such modules (Sect. 9.2) have promising results in further adapting the controller to the current state and activities of an individual by using various observation horizons of the recent past performance of the control system.

The multimodular structure presented in Fig. 1.2 illustrates the flexibility of adding new modules to an adaptive multivariable AP to address the challenges of low/high BGC, and the effects of MESS disturbances. As more powerful and data-intensive algorithms are added to the AP, the completion of all computations to provide the next insulin infusion flow rate in a timely manner becomes challenging. A layered architecture for executing various algorithms should be considered (Cinar 2017). The basic control activities should be computed in the computational capabilities housed in the pump system. This will provide uninterrupted control even when there are interruptions in communication. Additional AP control modules should be provided in a dedicated smartphone, and additional modules that necessitate execution of complex algorithms and access to large databases should be performed in cloud-based servers. Information safety and security (for data integrity and protection from malice) will be critical.

Much work is needed for making AP systems user-friendly for all populations (different age groups, comfort levels with technology, visual impairments, and other handicaps) affordable and intuitive. This will help acceptance both by people with

T1D and by the medical community that is turning over the responsibility of maintaining the BGC in the desirable range to an automated algorithm.

The creativity and pioneer spirit of individuals with T1D or their family member or friends have contributed to the development of technologies for improving the AP (diaTribe 2017; DiabetesMine 2017). Products such as do-it-yourself APs (diyps.org 2017), Nightscout CGM monitoring system, and Tidepool (2017) are used by many people. Industry and regulatory agencies have acted swiftly to evaluate and approve similar products. Various start-up companies are proposing novel AP technologies focusing of control algorithms (TypeZeroTechnologies 2017), algorithms and control devices (BetaBionics 2017), sensors and delivery systems (PacificDiabetesTechnologies 2017), and algorithms and insulin pumps (BigfootBiomedical 2017), to name a few of them. Several clinical trials are ongoing to test the AP concepts proposed and assess their performances in response to meal and exercise challenges (a representative list is available at ClinicalTrials.gov (2017)). This creativity, positive and collaborative attitude, and federal and private funding of T1D and AP research complement the advances in technology to provide a fertile environment to improve the AP systems and the quality of life of people with T1D.

References

Agamennoni G, Nieto JI, Nebot EM (2011) An outlier-robust Kalman filter. In: 2011 IEEE international conference on robotics and automation (ICRA). IEEE, pp 1551–1558

Agar BU, Eren M, Cinar A (2006) Glucosim: educational software for virtual experiments with patients with type 1 diabetes. In: IEEE-EMBS 27th annual international conference on engineering in medicine and biology society. IEEE, pp 845–848

Alberti KGMM, Zimmet PZ (1998) Definition, diagnosis and classification of diabetes mellitus and its complications. Part 1: diagnosis and classification of diabetes mellitus. Provisional report of a WHO Consultation. Diabetic Medicine 15(7):539–553

Albisser A, Leibel B, Ewart T, Davidovac Z, Botz C, Zingg W (1974) An artificial endocrine pancreas. Diabetes 23(5):389–396

Andre D, Pelletier R, Farringdon J, Safier S, Talbott W, Stone R, Vyas N, Trimble J, Wolf D, Vishnubhatla S, et al (2006) The development of the sensewear® armband, a revolutionary energy assessment device to assess physical activity and lifestyle. BodyMedia Inc

Åström KJ, Hägglund T (2006) Advanced PID control. ISA-The instrumentation, systems and automation society

Atlas E, Nimri R, Miller S, Grunberg EA, Phillip M (2010) MD-logic artificial pancreas system a pilot study in adults with type 1 diabetes. Diabetes Care 33(5):1072–1076

Badwe AS, Singh A, Patwardhan SC, Gudi RD (2010) A constrained recursive pseudo-linear regression scheme for on-line parameter estimation in adaptive control. J Process Control 20(5):559–572

Bakhtiani PA, Zhao LM, El Youssef J, Castle JR, Ward WK (2013) A review of artificial pancreas technologies with an emphasis on bi-hormonal therapy. Diabetes Obes Metab 15(12):1065–1070

Bally L, Thabit H, Kojzar H, Mader JK, Qerimi-Hyseni J, Hartnell S, Tauschmann M, Allen JM, Wilinska ME, Pieber TR et al (2017) Day-and-night glycaemic control with closed-coop insulin delivery versus conventional insulin pump therapy in free-living adults with well controlled type 1 diabetes: an open-label, randomised, crossover study. Lancet Diabetes Endocrinol 5(4):261–270

Bantle JP, Wylie-Rosett J, Albright AL, Apovian CM, Clark NG, Franz MJ, Hoogwerf BJ, Lichtenstein AH, Mayer-Davis E, Mooradian AD et al (2008) Nutrition recommendations and interventions for diabetes: a position statement of the American Diabetes Association. Diabetes Care 31:S61–S78

Barnard K, James J, Kerr D, Adolfsson P, Runion A, Serbedzija G (2016) Impact of chronic sleep disturbance for people living with type 1 diabetes. J Diabetes Sci Technol 10(3):762–767

A. Cinar and K. Turksoy, *Advances in Artificial Pancreas Systems*,
SpringerBriefs in Bioengineering, https://doi.org/10.1007/978-3-319-72245-0

Baucom KJ, Queen TL, Wiebe DJ, Turner SL, Wolfe KL, Godbey EI, Fortenberry KT, Mansfield JH, Berg CA (2015) Depressive symptoms, daily stress, and adherence in late adolescents with type 1 diabetes. Health Psychol 34(5):522

Bayrak ES, Turksoy K, Cinar A, Quinn L, Littlejohn E, Rollins D et al (2012) Hypoglycemia early alarm systems based on recursive autoregressive partial least squares models. J Diabetes Sci Technol 7(1):206–214

Baysal N, Cameron F, Buckingham BA, Wilson DM, Bequette BW (2013) Detecting Sensor and insulin infusion set anomalies in an artificial pancreas. In: American control conference (ACC). IEEE, pp 2929–2933

Baysal N, Cameron F, Buckingham BA, Wilson DM, Chase HP, Maahs DM, Bequette BW, Aye T, Clinton P, Harris BP et al (2014) A novel method to detect pressure-induced sensor attenuations (PISA) in an artificial pancreas. J Diabetes Sci Technol 8(6):1091–1096

Beck RW, Raghinaru D, Wadwa RP, Chase HP, Maahs DM, Buckingham BA et al (2014) Frequency of morning ketosis after overnight insulin suspension using an automated nocturnal predictive low glucose suspend system. Diabetes Care 37(5):1224–1229

Bequette BW (2010) Continuous glucose monitoring: real-time algorithms for calibration, filtering, and alarms. J Diabetes Sci Technol 4(2):404–418

Bergenstal RM, Tamborlane WV, Ahmann A, Buse JB, Dailey G, Davis SN, Joyce C, Peoples T, Perkins BA, Welsh JB, et al (2010) Effectiveness of sensor-augmented insulin-pump therapy in type 1 diabetes. New Engl J Med 363(4):311–320

Bergman RN (1989) Toward physiological understanding of glucose tolerance: minimal-model approach. Diabetes 38(12):1512–1527

Bergman RN, Ider YZ, Bowden CR, Cobelli C (1979) Quantitative estimation of insulin sensitivity. Am J Physiol Endocrinol Metab 236(6):E667

Bergman RN, Phillips LS, Cobelli C (1981) Physiologic evaluation of factors controlling glucose tolerance in man: measurement of insulin sensitivity and beta-cell glucose sensitivity from the response to intravenous glucose. J Clin Investig 68(6):1456

Berndt DJ, Clifford J (1994) Using dynamic time warping to find patterns in time series. Knowledge discovery and data mining workshop. Seattle, WA, pp 359–370

BetaBionics (2017). https://www.betabionics.org

BigfootBiomedical (2017). https://www.bigfootbiomedical.com/first-clinical-trial/

Blauw H, van Bon A, Koops R, DeVries J (2016) Performance and safety of an integrated bihormonal artificial pancreas for fully automated glucose control at home. Diabetes Obes Metab 18(7):671–677

Bliss M (2013) The discovery of insulin. University Of Chicago Press

van Bon AC, Hermanides J, Koops R, Hoekstra JB, DeVries JH (2010) Postprandial glycemic excursions with the use of a closed-loop platform in subjects with type 1 diabetes: a pilot study. J Diabetes Sci Technol 4(4):923–928

van Bon AC, Luijf YM, Koebrugge R, Koops R, Hoekstra JB, DeVries JH (2014) Feasibility of a portable bihormonal closed-loop system to control glucose excursions at home under free-living conditions for 48 hours. Diabetes Technol Ther 16(3):131–136

Bondia J, Tarín C, García-Gabin W, Esteve E, Fernández-Real JM, Ricart W, Vehí J (2008) Using support vector machines to detect therapeutically incorrect measurements by the MiniMed CGMS. J Diabetes Sci Technol 2(4):622–629

Breton M, Farret A, Bruttomesso D, Anderson S, Magni L, Patek S, Dalla Man C, Place J, Demartini S, Del Favero S et al (2012) Fully integrated artificial pancreas in type 1 diabetes modular closed-loop glucose control maintains near normoglycemia. Diabetes 61(9):2230–2237

Breton MD, Brown SA, Karvetski CH, Kollar L, Topchyan KA, Anderson SM, Kovatchev BP (2014) Adding heart rate signal to a control-to-range artificial pancreas system improves the protection against hypoglycemia during exercise in type 1 diabetes. Diabetes Technol Therap 16(8):506–511

Breton MD, Cherñavvsky DR, Forlenza GP, DeBoer MD, Robic J, Wadwa RP, Messer LH, Kovatchev BP, Maahs DM (2017) Closed loop control during intense prolonged outdoor exercise in adolescents with type 1 diabetes: the artificial pancreas Ski Study. Diabetes Care 1:1. https://doi.org/10.2337/dc17-0883

Brown SA, Breton MD, Anderson S, Kollar L, Levy C, Lam D, Levister C, Kudva YC, Basu A, Mccrady-Spitzer S et al (2015) Artificial pancreas improves glycemic control in a Multi-night Multicenter Outpatient/home study of patients with T1D. Diabetes Am Diabetes Assoc 64:A59–A59

Buckingham B, Cobry E, Clinton P, Gage V, Caswell K, Kunselman E, Cameron F, Chase HP (2009) Preventing hypoglycemia using predictive alarm algorithms and insulin pump suspension. Diabetes Technol Therap 11(2):93–97

Buckingham B, Chase HP, Dassau E, Cobry E, Clinton P, Gage V, Caswell K, Wilkinson J, Cameron F, Lee H et al (2010) Prevention of nocturnal hypoglycemia using predictive alarm algorithms and insulin pump suspension. Diabetes Care 33(5):1013–1017

Buckingham BA, Raghinaru D, Cameron F, Bequette BW, Chase HP, Maahs DM, Slover R, Wadwa RP, Wilson DM, Ly T et al (2015) Predictive low-glucose insulin suspension reduces duration of nocturnal hypoglycemia in children without increasing ketosis. Diabetes Care 38(7):1197–1204

Cameron F, Niemeyer G, Buckingham BA (2009) Probabilistic evolving meal detection and estimation of meal total glucose appearance. J Diabetes Sci Technol 3(5):1022–1030

Cameron F, Niemeyer G, Bequette BW (2012a) Extended multiple model prediction with application to blood glucose regulation. J Process Control 22(8):1422–1432

Cameron F, Wilson DM, Buckingham BA, Arzumanyan H, Clinton P, Chase HP, Lum J, Maahs DM, Calhoun PM, Bequette BW (2012b) Inpatient studies of a Kalman-filter-based predictive pump shutoff algorithm. J Diabetes Sci Technol 6(5):1142–1147

Campetelli G, Zumoffen D, Basualdo M (2011) Improvements on noninvasive blood glucose biosensors using wavelets for quick fault detection. J Sens 2011

Carson E, Cobelli C (2014) Modelling methodology for physiology and medicine, 2nd edn. Elsevier

Castle JR, Engle JM, El Youssef J, Massoud RG, Yuen KC, Kagan R, Ward WK (2010) Novel use of glucagon in a closed-loop system for prevention of hypoglycemia in type 1 diabetes. Diabetes Care 33(6):1282–1287

Caumo A, Vicini P, Zachwieja JJ, Avogaro A, Yarasheski K, Bier DM, Cobelli C (1999) Undermodeling affects minimal model indexes: insights from a two-compartment model. Am J Physiol Endocrinol Metab 276(6):E1171–E1193

Cengiz E (2013) Closer to ideal insulin action: ultra fast acting insulins. Panminerva Medica 55(3):269–275

Cengiz E, Sherr JL, Weinzimer SA, Tamborlane WV (2011) New-generation diabetes management: glucose sensor-augmented insulin pump therapy. Expert Rev Med Devices 8(4):449–458

Cengiz E, Weinzimer SA, Sherr JL, Tichy E, Martin M, Carria L, Steffen A, Tamborlane WV (2013) Acceleration of insulin pharmacodynamic profile by a novel insulin infusion site warming device. Pediatr Diabetes 14(3):168–173

Cengiz E, Weinzimer SA, Sherr JL, Tichy EM, Carria L, Cappiello D, Steffen A, Tamborlane WV (2014) Faster in and faster out: accelerating insulin absorption and action by insulin infusion site warming. Diabetes Technol Therap 16(1):20–25

Centers for Disease Control and Prevention (2011) National diabetes fact sheet: national estimates and general information on diabetes and prediabetes in the United States, 2011. US Department of Health and Human Services

Centers for Disease Control and Prevention (2012) Number of emergency department visits (in Thousands) with hyperglycemic crisis as first-listed diagnosis, All ages, United States, 2006–2009. https://www.cdc.gov/diabetes/statistics/hyperglycemia/fig1.htm

Centers for Disease Control and Prevention (2014) Number of emergency department visits (In Thousands) with hypoglycemia as first-listed diagnosis and diabetes as secondary diagnosis, Adults aged 18 years or older, United States, 2006–2009. https://www.cdc.gov/diabetes/statistics/hypoglycemia/fig1.htm

Centers for Disease Control and Prevention and Others (2014) National diabetes statistics report: estimates of diabetes and its burden in the United States. US Department of Health and Human services 2014

Chakrabarty A, Zavitsanou S, Doyle III F, Dassau E (2017) Event-triggered model predictive control for embedded artificial pancreas systems. IEEE Trans Biomed Eng

Chee F, Fernando T (2001) Closed-loop control of blood glucose. Springer

Chida Y, Hamer M (2008) An association of adverse psychosocial factors with diabetes mellitus: a meta-analytic review of longitudinal cohort studies

Cichosz SL, Frystyk J, Hejlesen OK, Tarnow L, Fleischer J (2014) A novel algorithm for prediction and detection of hypoglycemia based on continuous glucose monitoring and heart rate variability in patients with type 1 diabetes. J Diabetes Sci Technol 8(4):731–737

Cinar A (2017) Multivariable adaptive artificial pancreas system in type 1 diabetes. Curr Diabetes Rep 17(10):88

Cinar A, Palazoglu A, Kayihan F (2007) Chemical process performance evaluation. CRC Press

Clarke D, Mohtadi C, Tuffs P (1987a) Generalized predictive controlpart I. The basic algorithm. Automatica 23(2):137–148

Clarke D, Mohtadi C, Tuffs P (1987b) Generalized predictive controlpart II extensions and interpretations. Automatica 23(2):149–160

Clarke DW, Mohtadi C (1989) Properties of generalized predictive control. Automatica 25(6):859–875

Cleveland WS (1979) Robust locally weighted regression and smoothing scatterplots. J Am Stat Assoc 74(368):829–836

ClinicalDiabetesgov (2017). https://clinicaltrials.gov/ct2/results?term=artificial+pancreas&cond=Diabetes&Search=Apply&recrs=a&recrs=d&age_v=&gndr=&type=&rslt=

Cobelli C, Mari A (1983) Validation of mathematical models of complex endocrine-metabolic systems. a case study on a model of glucose regulation. Med Biol Eng Comput 21(4):390–399

Cobelli C, Federspil G, Pacini G, Salvan A, Scandellari C (1982) An integrated mathematical model of the dynamics of blood glucose and its hormonal control. Math Biosci 58(1):27–60

Cobelli C, Pacini G, Toffolo G, Sacca L (1986) Estimation of insulin sensitivity and glucose clearance from minimal model: new insights from labeled IVGTT. Am J Physiol Endocrinol Metab 250(5):E591–E598

Cobelli C, Caumo A, Omenetto M (1999) Minimal model SG overestimation and SI underestimation: improved accuracy by a Bayesian two-compartment model. Am J Physiol Endocrinol Metab 277(3):E481–E488

Cohen ND, Hong ES, Van Drie C, Balkau B, Shaw J (2013) Long-term metabolic effects of continuous subcutaneous insulin infusion therapy in type 1 diabetes. Diabetes Technol Therap 15(7):544–549

Colberg SR, Edelman SV (2008) 50 secrets of the longest living people with diabetes. Da Capo Press

Collier G, McLean A, O'dea K, (1984) Effect of co-ingestion of fat on the metabolic responses to slowly and rapidly absorbed carbohydrates. Diabetologia 26(1):50–54

Cryer PE, Davis SN, Shamoon H (2003) Hypoglycemia in diabetes. Diabetes Care 26(6):1902–1912

Dalla Man C, Micheletto F, Lv D, Breton M, Kovatchev B, Cobelli C (2014) The UVA/Padova type 1 diabetes simulator new features. J Diabetes Sci Technol 8(1):26–34

Damiano ER, El-Khatib FH, Zheng H, Nathan DM, Russell SJ (2013) A comparative effectiveness analysis of three continuous glucose monitors. Diabetes Care 36(2):251–259

Damiano ER, McKeon K, El-Khatib FH, Zheng H, Nathan DM, Russell SJ (2014) A comparative effectiveness analysis of three continuous glucose monitors: the Navigator, G4 Platinum, and Enlite. J Diabetes Sci Technol 8(4):699–708

Dasanayake IS, Bevier WC, Castorino K, Pinsker JE, Seborg DE, Doyle FJ III, Dassau E (2015) Early detection of physical activity for people with type 1 diabetes mellitus. J Diabetes Sci Technol 9(6):1236–1245

Dassau E, Bequette BW, Buckingham BA, Doyle FJ (2008) Detection of a meal using continuous glucose monitoring implications for an artificial β-cell. Diabetes Care 31(2):295–300

Dassau E, Cameron F, Lee H, Bequette BW, Zisser H, Jovanovič L, Chase HP, Wilson DM, Buckingham BA, Doyle FJ (2010) Real-time hypoglycemia prediction suite using continuous glucose monitoring a safety net for the artificial pancreas. Diabetes Care 33(6):1249–1254

DCCT Research Group and Others (1991) Epidemiology of severe hypoglycemia in the diabetes control and complications trial. Am J Med 90(4):450–459

De Gaetano A, Arino O (2000) Mathematical modelling of the intravenous glucose tolerance test. J Math Biol 40(2):136–168

Deiss D, Bolinder J, Riveline JP, Battelino T, Bosi E, Tubiana-Rufi N, Kerr D, Phillip M (2006) Improved glycemic control in poorly controlled patients with type 1 diabetes using real-time continuous glucose monitoring. Diabetes Care 29(12):2730–2732

Del Favero S, Monaro M, Facchinetti A, Tagliavini A, Sparacino G, Cobelli C (2014) Real-time detection of Glucose Sensor snd Insulin Pump Faults in an artificial pancreas. IFAC Proc 47(3):1941–1946

Dempster AP, Laird NM, Rubin DB (1977) Maximum likelihood from incomplete data via the EM algorithm. J R Stati Soc Ser B (Methodol) 1–38

Dexcom (2016) Dexcom share. http://www.dexcom.com/dexcom-share

Diabetes atlas (2014) International Diabetes Federation

Diabetes Research in Children Network (DirecNet) Study group and others (2008) The accuracy of the guardian® RT Continuous glucose monitorn children with type 1 diabetes. Diabetes Technol Therap 10(4):266–272

DiabetesMine (2017). http://www.healthline.com/diabetesmine

diaTribe (2017). https://diatribe.org

diypsorg (2017). https://diyps.org/2014/02/07/a-diy-artificial-pancreas-systemurl

Downie P (2013) Practical aspects of capillary blood glucose monitoring: a simple guide for primary care. Diabetes Prim Care 15:149–153

Doyle FJ, Huyett LM, Lee JB, Zisser HC, Dassau E (2014) Closed-loop artificial pancreas systems: engineering the algorithms. Diabetes Care 37(5):1191–1197

Edelman SV (2007) When glucose levels are too low: a major barrier to taking control of your diabetes. Insulin 2(2):99–101

El-Khatib FH, Russell SJ, Nathan DM, Sutherlin RG, Damiano ER (2010) A bihormonal closed-loop artificial pancreas for type 1 diabetes. Sci Trans Med 2(27):27ra27–27ra27

El-Khatib FH, Russell SJ, Magyar KL, Sinha M, McKeon K, Nathan DM, Damiano ER (2014) Autonomous and continuous adaptation of a bihormonal bionic pancreas in adults and adolescents with type 1 diabetes. J Clin Endocrinol Metab 99(5):1701–1711

Elleri D, Maltoni G, Allen JM, Nodale M, Kumareswaran K, Leelarathna L, Thabit H, Caldwell K, Wilinska ME, Calhoun P, Kollman C, Dunger DB, Hovorka R (2014) Safety of closed-loop therapy during reduction or omission of meal boluses in adolescents with type 1 diabetes: a randomized clinical trial. Diabetes Obes Metab 16(11):1174–1178

Eren M, Agar B, Erzen F, Cinar A (2005) GlucoSim: A web-based educational simulation package for glucose-insulin levels in the human body. http://simulator.iit.edu/web/glucosim/index.html

Eren-Oruklu M, Cinar A, Quinn L, Smith D (2009) Estimation of future glucose concentrations with subject-specific recursive linear models. Diabetes Technol Therap 11(4):243–253

Eren-Oruklu M, Cinar A, Quinn L (2010) Hypoglycemia prediction with subject-specific recursive time-series models. J Diabetes Sci Technol 4(1):25–33

Estrada CL, Danielson KK, Drum ML, Lipton RB (2012) Insufficient sleep in young patients with diabetes and their families. Biol Res Nurs 14(1):48–54

Facchinetti A, Del Favero S, Sparacino G, Cobelli C (2011) Detecting failures of the glucose sensor-insulin pump system: improved overnight safety monitoring for type-1 diabetes. In: EMBC, annual international conference of the IEEE engineering in medicine and biology society. IEEE, pp 4947–4950

Facchinetti A, Favero S, Sparacino G, Cobelli C (2013) An online failure detection method of the glucose sensor-insulin pump system: improved overnight safety of type-1 diabetic subjects. IEEE Trans Biomed Eng 60(2):406–416

Facchinetti A, Del Favero S, Sparacino G, Cobelli C (2016) Modeling transient disconnections and compression artifacts of continuous glucose sensors. Diabetes Technol Therap 18(4):264–272

Feng J, Turksoy K, Cinar A (2016a) Performance assessment of model-based artificial pancreas control systems. In: Prediction methods for blood glucose concentration. Springer, pp 243–265

Feng J, Turksoy K, Samadi S, Hajizadeh I, Cinar A (2016b) Hybrid online sensor error detection and functional redundancy for artificial pancreas control systems. IFAC-PapersOnLine 49(7):753–758

Feng J, Turksoy K, Samadi S, Hajizadeh I, Littlejohn E, Cinar A (2017) Hybrid online sensor error detection and functional redundancy for systems with time-varying parameters. J Process Control. https://doi.org/10.1016/j.jprocont.2017.04.004

Feng J, Hajizadeh I, Yu X, Rashid M, Turksoy K, Samadi S, Sevil M, Frantz N, Brandt R, Lazaro C, Maloney Z, Littlejohn E, Philipson L, Gannon G, Cinar A (2018) Multi-level supervision and modification for artificial pancreas control system. Comput Chem Eng 112:57–69

Feupe SF, Frias PF, Mednick SC, McDevitt EA, Heintzman ND (2013) Nocturnal continuous glucose and sleep stage data in adults with type 1 diabetes in real-world conditions. J Diabetes Sci Technol 7(5):1337–1345

Forlenza G, Chernavvsky D, DeBoer M, Robic J, Kovatchev B, Wadwa P, Messel L, Maahs D, Breton M (2017) The artificial pancreas improves glycemic control during extended exercise at ski camp in adolescents with type 1 diabetes. Diabetes Technol Therap 19:A–47

Franz MJ, Bantle JP, Beebe CA, Brunzell JD, Chiasson JL, Garg A, Holzmeister LA, Hoogwerf B, Mayer-Davis E, Mooradian AD et al (2002) Evidence-based nutrition principles and recommendations for the treatment and prevention of diabetes and related complications. Diabetes Care 25(1):148–198

Frenzel MP, McCaul KD, Glasgow RE, Schafer LC (1988) The relationship of stress and coping to regimen adherence and glycemic control of diabetes. J Soc Clin Psychol 6(1):77–87

Frost G, Brynes A, Dhillo W, Bloom S, McBurney M (2003) The effects of fiber enrichment of pasta and fat content on gastric emptying, GLP-1, glucose, and insulin responses to a meal. Eur J Clin Nutr 57(2):293–298

Galassetti P, Riddell MC (2013) Exercise and type 1 tiabetes (T1DM). Compr Physiol 3(3):1309–36

Gani A, Gribok AV, Rajaraman S, Ward WK, Reifman J (2009) Predicting subcutaneous glucose concentration in humans: data-driven glucose modeling. IEEE Trans Biomed Eng 56(2):246–254

Garg S, Brazg RL, Bailey TS, Buckingham BA, Slover RH, Klonoff DC, Shin J, Welsh JB, Kaufman FR (2012) Reduction in duration of hypoglycemia by automatic suspension of insulin delivery: the in-clinic ASPIRE study. Diabetes Technol Therap 14(3):205–209

Ghahramani Z, Beal M (2000) Graphical models and variational methods. In: Saad D, Opper M (eds) Advanced mean field methods–theory and practice

Ghosal S, Nunley A, Mahbod P, Lewis AG, Smith EP, Tong J, D'Alessio DA, Herman JP (2015) Mouse handling limits the impact of stress on metabolic endpoints. Physiol Behav 150:31–37

Ginsberg BH (2009) Factors affecting blood glucose monitoring: sources of errors in measurement. J Diabetes Sci Technol 3(4):903–913

Golicki D, Golicka D, Groele L, Pankowska E (2008) Continuous Glucose Monitoring System in children with type 1 diabetes mellitus: a systematic review and meta-analysis. Diabetologia 51(2):233–240

Gonder-Frederick LA, Carter WR, Cox DJ, Clarke WL (1990) Environmental stress and blood glucose change in insulin-dependent diabetes mellitus. Health Psychol 9(5):503

Gonder-Frederick LA, Grabman JH, Kovatchev B, Brown SA, Patek S, Basu A, Pinsker JE, Kudva YC, Wakeman CA, Dassau E et al (2016) Is psychological stress a factor for incorporation into future closed-loop systems? J Diabetes Sci Technol 10(3):640–646

Gondhalekar R, Dassau E, Doyle FJ (2016) Periodic zone-MPC with asymmetric costs for outpatient-ready safety of an artificial pancreas to treat type 1 diabetes. Automatica 71:237–246

Guerci B, Floriot M, Böhme P, Durain D, Benichou M, Jellimann S, Drouin P (2003) Clinical performance of CGMS in type 1 diabetic patients treated by continuous subcutaneous insulin infusion using insulin analogs. Diabetes Care 26(3):582–589

Hägglund T (1999) Automatic detection of sluggish control loops. Control Eng Pract 7(12):1505–1511

Haidar A, Legault L, Dallaire M, Alkhateeb A, Coriati A, Messier V, Cheng P, Millette M, Boulet B, Rabasa-Lhoret R (2013) Glucose-responsive insulin and glucagon delivery (dual-hormone artificial pancreas) in adults with type 1 diabetes: a randomized crossover controlled trial. Can Med Assoc J 185(4):297–305

Haidar A, Farid D, St-Yves A, Messier V, Chen V, Xing D, Brazeau AS, Duval C, Boulet B, Legault L et al (2014) Post-breakfast closed-loop glucose control is improved when accompanied with carbohydrate-matching bolus compared to weight-dependent bolus. Diabetes Metab 40(3):211–214

Hajizadeh I, Rashid MM, Turksoy K, Samadi S, Feng J, Frantz N, Sevil M, Cengiz E, Cinar A (2017) Plasma insulin estimation in people with type 1 diabetes mellitus. Ind Eng Chem Res 56(35):9846–9857

Halford W, Cuddihy S, Mortimer R (1990) Psychological stress and blood glucose regulation in type 1 diabetic patients. Health Psychol 9(5):516

Halimi S (2010) Acute consequences of hypoglycaemia in diabetic patients. Diabetes Metab 36:S75–S83

Hanas R, Ragnar Hanas M (2009) Type 1 diabetes in children, adolescents and young adults, 4th edn. Class Publication, Class Health

Hanson SL, Pichert JW (1986) Perceived stress and diabetes control in adolescents. Health Psychol 5(5):439

Hart P (1968) The condensed nearest neighbor rule (Corresp.). IEEE Trans Inf Theory 14(3):515–516

Hegenbarth MA et al (2008) Preparing for pediatric emergencies: drugs to consider. Pediatrics 121(2):433–443

Heinemann L, Muchmore DB (2012) Ultrafast-acting insulins: state of the art. J Diabetes Sci Technol 6(4):728–742

Hilliard ME, Joyce P, Hessler D, Butler AM, Anderson BJ, Jaser S (2016) Stress and A1c among people with diabetes across the lifespan. Current Diabetes Rep 16(8):1–10

Holt RI, Cockram C, Flyvbjerg A, Goldstein BJ (2011) Textbook of diabetes. Wiley

Holt S, Carter D, Tothill P, Heading R, Prescott L (1979) Effect of gel fibre on gastric emptying and absorption of glucose and paracetamol. Lancet 313(8117):636–639

Hovorka R, Shojaee-Moradie F, Carroll PV, Chassin LJ, Gowrie IJ, Jackson NC, Tudor RS, Umpleby AM, Jones RH (2002) Partitioning glucose distribution/transport, disposal, and endogenous production during IVGTT. Am J Physiol Endocrinol Metab 282(5):E992–E1007

Hovorka R, Canonico V, Chassin LJ, Haueter U, Massi-Benedetti M, Federici MO, Pieber TR, Schaller HC, Schaupp L, Vering T et al (2004) Nonlinear model predictive control of glucose concentration in subjects with type 1 diabetes. Physiol Meas 25(4):905–920

Hovorka R, Allen JM, Elleri D, Chassin LJ, Harris J, Xing D, Kollman C, Hovorka T, Larsen AMF, Nodale M et al (2010) Manual closed-loop insulin delivery in children and adolescents with type 1 diabetes: a phase 2 randomised crossover trial. Lancet 375(9716):743–751

Howey DC, Bowsher RR, Brunelle RL, Woodworth JR (1994) [Lys (B28), Pro (B29)]-human insulin: a rapidly absorbed analogue of human insulin. Diabetes 43(3):396–402

Hughes CS, Patek SD, Breton MD, Kovatchev BP (2010) Hypoglycemia prevention via pump attenuation and red-yellow-green traffic lights using continuous glucose monitoring and insulin pump data. J Diabetes Sci Technol 4(5):1146–1155

Jacobs PG, El Youssef J, Castle J, Bakhtiani P, Branigan D, Breen M, Bauer D, Preiser N, Leonard G, Stonex T et al (2014) Automated control of an adaptive bihormonal, dual-sensor artificial pancreas and evaluation during inpatient studies. IEEE Trans Biomed Eng 61(10):2569–2581

Jaser SS, Ellis D (2016) Sleep in adolescents and young adults with type 1 diabetes: associations with diabetes management and glycemic control. Health Psychol Behav Med 4(1):49–55

Jauch-Chara K, Schmid SM, Hallschmid M, Born J, Schultes B (2008) Altered neuroendocrine sleep architecture in patients with type 1 diabetes. Diabetes Care 31(6):1183–1188

Jenkins D, Wolever T, Leeds AR, Gassull MA, Haisman P, Dilawari J, Goff DV, Metz GL, Alberti K (1978) Dietary fibres, fibre analogues, and glucose tolerance: importance of viscosity. Br Med J 1(6124):1392–1394

Jenkins D, Wolever T, Taylor RH, Barker H, Fielden H, Baldwin JM, Bowling AC, Newman HC, Jenkins AL, Goff DV (1981) Glycemic index of foods: a physiological basis for carbohydrate exchange. Am J Clin Nutr 34(3):362–366

Julier SJ, Uhlmann JK (2004) Unscented filtering and nonlinear estimation. Proc IEEE 92(3):401–422

Juvenile Diabetes Research Foundation Continuous Glucose Monitoring Study Group and Others (2008) Continuous glucose monitoring and intensive treatment of type 1 diabetes. New Engl J Med 2008(359):1464–1476

Kajantie E, Phillips DI (2006) The effects of sex and hormonal status on the physiological response to acute psychosocial stress. Psychoneuroendocrinology 31(2):151–178

Kandepu R, Foss B, Imsland L (2008) Applying the unscented Kalman filter for nonlinear state estimation. J Process Control 18(7):753–768

Kanderian SS, Weinzimer S, Voskanyan G, Steil GM (2009) Identification of intraday metabolic profiles during closed-loop glucose control in individuals with type 1 diabetes. J Diabetes Sci Technol 3(5):1047–1057

Kanderian Jr SS, Steil GM (2010) Apparatus and method for controlling insulin infusion with state variable feedback. US Patent 7,806,886

Kelly MM, Tyrka AR, Anderson GM, Price LH, Carpenter LL (2008) Sex differences in emotional and physiological responses to the Trier Social Stress Test. J Behav Therapy Exp Psychiatry 39(1):87–98

Keogh EJ, Pazzani MJ (2001) Derivative dynamic time warping. In: Proceedings of the 2001 SIAM international conference on data mining, SIAM, vol 1, pp 5–7

Kim S, Okajima R, Kano M, Hasebe S (2013) Development of soft-sensor using locally weighted PLS with adaptive similarity measure. Chemom Intell Lab Syst 124:43–49

Klonoff DC (2005) Continuous glucose monitoring roadmap for 21st century diabetes therapy. Diabetes Care 28(5):1231–1239

Klonoff DC, Zimliki CL, Stevens LA, Beaston P, Pinkos A, Choe SY, Arreaza-Rubín G, Heetderks W (2011) Innovations in technology for the treatment of diabetes: clinical development of the artificial pancreas (an autonomous system)

Knobbe EJ, Buckingham B (2005) The extended Kalman filter for continuous glucose monitoring. Diabetes Technol Therap 7(1):15–27

Koren D, OSullivan KL, Mokhlesi B, (2015) Metabolic and glycemic sequelae of sleep disturbances in children and adults. Current Diabetes Rep 15(1):562

Kovatchev B, Breton M, Dalla Man C, Cobelli C (2008) In silico model and computer simulation environment approximating the human glucose/insulin utilization. Food and drug administration master file MAF 1521

Kowalski A (2015) Pathway to artificial pancreas systems revisited: moving downstream. Diabetes Care 38(6):1036–1043

Kowalski A, Lum JW (2009) Juvenile diabetes research foundation artificial pancreas consortium update. J Diabetes Sci Technol 3(5):1224–1226

Kropff J, Del Favero S, Place J, Toffanin C, Visentin R, Monaro M, Messori M, Di Palma F, Lanzola G, Farret A et al (2015) 2 month evening and night closed-loop glucose control in patients with type 1 diabetes under free-living conditions: a randomised crossover trial. Lancet Diabetes Endocrinol 3(12):939–947

Kudva YC, Carter RE, Cobelli C, Basu R, Basu A (2014) Closed-loop artificial pancreas systems: physiological input to enhance next-generation devices. Diabetes Care 37(5):1184–1190

Kumareswaran K, Elleri D, Allen JM, Harris J, Xing D, Kollman C, Nodale M, Murphy HR, Amiel SA, Heller SR et al (2011) Meta-analysis of overnight closed-loop randomized studies in children and adults with type 1 diabetes: the Cambridge cohort. J Diabetes Sci Technol 5(6):1352–1362

Lacy SL, Bernstein DS (2002) Subspace identification with guaranteed stability using constrained optimization. Am Control Conf (ACC) 4:3307–3312

Lacy SL, Bernstein DS (2003) Subspace identification with guaranteed stability using constrained optimization. IEEE Trans Autom Control 48(7):1259–1263

Leal Y, Gonzalez-Abril L, Lorencio C, Bondia J, Vehi J (2013a) Detection of correct and incorrect measurements in real-time continuous glucose monitoring systems by applying a postprocessing support vector machine. IEEE Trans Biomed Eng 60(7):1891–1899

Leal Y, Ruiz M, Lorencio C, Bondia J, Mujica L, Vehi J (2013b) Principal component analysis in combination with case-based reasoning for detecting therapeutically correct and incorrect measurements in continuous glucose monitoring systems. Biomed Signal Process Control 8(6):603–614

Lee H, Buckingham BA, Wilson DM, Bequette BW (2009) A closed-loop artificial pancreas using model predictive control and a sliding meal size estimator. J Diabetes Sci Technol 3(5):1082–1090

Lehmann E, Deutsch T (1992) A physiological model of glucose-insulin interaction in type 1 diabetes mellitus. J Biomed Eng 14(3):235–242

Lenhard MJ, Reeves GD (2001) Continuous subcutaneous insulin infusion: a comprehensive review of insulin pump therapy. Arch Intern Med 161(19):2293–2300

Liebl A, Hoogma R, Renard E, Geelhoed-Duijvestijn P, Klein E, Diglas J, Kessler L, Melki V, Diem P, Brun JM et al (2009) A reduction in severe hypoglycaemia in type 1 diabetes in a randomized crossover study of continuous intraperitoneal compared with subcutaneous insulin infusion. Diabetes Obes Metab 11(11):1001–1008

Ljung L (1979) Asymptotic behavior of the extended Kalman filter as a parameter estimator for linear systems. IEEE Trans Autom Control 24(1):36–50

Lyashevskiy S, Chen Y (1997) The lyapunov stability theory in system identification. Am Control Conf 1:617–621 (IEEE)

Magni L, Forgione M, Toffanin C, Dalla Man C, Kovatchev B, De Nicolao G, Cobelli C (2009) Run-to-run tuning of model predictive control for type 1 diabetes subjects: In Silico trial

Marcovecchio ML, Chiarelli F (2012) The effects of acute and chronic stress on diabetes control. Sci Signal 5(247):pt10–pt10

Mauseth R, Hirsch IB, Bollyky J, Kircher R, Matheson D, Sanda S, Greenbaum C (2013) Use of a fuzzy logi controller in a closed-loop artificial pancreas. Diabetes Technol Therap 15(8):628–633

Mauseth R, Lord SM, Hirsch IB, Kircher RC, Matheson DP, Greenbaum CJ (2015) Stress testing of an artificial pancreas system with pizza and exercise leads to improvements in the systems fuzzy logic controller. J Diabetes Sci Technol 9(6):1253–1259

McCall A, Farhy L (2013) Treating type 1 diabetes: from strategies for insulin delivery to dual hormonal control. Minerva Endocrinol 38(2):145

McDonough RJ, Clements MA, DeLurgio SA, Patton SR (2017) Sleep duration and its impact on adherence in adolescents with type 1 diabetes mellitus. Pediatr Diabetes 18(4):262–270

Medtronic (2017) Medtronic minimed 670g. https://www.medtronicdiabetes.com/loop-blog/important-update-minimed-670g-availability-priority-access-program/

Mensh BD, Wisniewski NA, Neil BM, Burnett DR (2013) Susceptibility of interstitial continuous glucose monitor performance to sleeping position. J Diabetes Sci Technol 7(4):863–870

Michael B (1982) The Discovery Of Insulin. Textbook Of Diabetes 1:13–243

Moberg E, Kollind M, Lins PE, Adamson U (1994) Acute mental stress impairs insulin sensitivity in IDDM patients. Diabetologia 37(3):247–251

Morrow L, Muchmore DB, Hompesch M, Ludington EA, Vaughn DE (2013) Comparative pharmacokinetics and insulin action for three rapid-acting insulin analogs injected subcutaneously with and without hyaluronidase. Diabetes Care 36(2):273–275

Mudaliar SR, Lindberg FA, Joyce M, Beerdsen P, Strange P, Lin A, Henry RR (1999) Insulin aspart (B28 ASP-insulin): a fast-acting analog of human insulin: absorption kinetics and action profile compared with regular human insulin in healthy nondiabetic subjects. Diabetes Care 22(9):1501–1506

Murphy HR, Kumareswaran K, Elleri D, Allen JM, Caldwell K, Biagioni M, Simmons D, Dunger DB, Nodale M, Wilinska ME et al (2011) Safety and efficacy of 24-h closed-loop insulin delivery in well-controlled pregnant women with type 1 diabetes a randomized crossover case series. Diabetes Care 34(12):2527–2529

National Institute of Diabetes and Digestive and Kidney Diseases (2016) Diabetes in America, 3rd edn. National Institutes of Health

Nelles O (2013) Nonlinear system identification: from classical approaches to neural networks and fuzzy models. Springer Science & Business Media

Nimri R, Atlas E, Ajzensztejn M, Miller S, Oron T, Phillip M (2012) Feasibility study of automated overnight closed-loop glucose control under md-logic artificial pancreas in patients with type 1 diabetes: the DREAM project. Diabetes Technol Therap 14(8):728–735

Nimri R, Muller I, Atlas E, Miller S, Fogel A, Bratina N, Kordonouri O, Battelino T, Danne T, Phillip M (2014a) MD-Logic overnight control for 6 weeks of home use in patients with type 1 diabetes: randomized crossover trial. Diabetes Care 37(11):3025–3032

Nimri R, Muller I, Atlas E, Miller S, Kordonouri O, Bratina N, Tsioli C, Stefanija MA, Danne T, Battelino T et al (2014b) Night glucose control with MD-Logic artificial pancreas in home setting: a single blind, randomized crossover trial-interim analysis. Pediatr Diabetes 15(2):91–99

Nuttall FQ, Mooradian AD, Gannon MC, Billington C, Krezowski P (1984) Effect of protein ingestion on the glucose and insulin response to a standardized oral glucose load. Diabetes Care 7(5):465–470

O'Connell M, Donath S, O'Neal D, Colman P, Ambler G, Jones T, Davis E, Cameron F (2009) Glycaemic impact of patient-led use of sensor-guided pump therapy in type 1 diabetes: a randomised controlled trial. Diabetologia 52(7):1250–1257

Ogunnaike BA (1994) Process dynamics, modeling, and control. Oxford University Press, Oxford

PacificDiabetesTechnologies (2017). http://pacificdt.com

Palerm C (2011) Physiologic insulin delivery with insulin feedback: a control systems perspective. Comput Methods Programs Biomed 102(2):130–137

Palerm CC, Bequette BW (2007) Hypoglycemia detection and prediction using continuous glucose monitoring-a study on hypoglycemic clamp data. J Diabetes Sci Technol 1(5):624–629

Palerm CC, Zisser H, Jovanovič L, Doyle FJ (2008) A run-to-run control strategy to adjust basal insulin infusion rates in type 1 diabetes. J Process Control 18(3):258–265

Patek SD, Magni L, Dassau E, Karvetski C, Toffanin C, De Nicolao G, Del Favero S, Breton M, Dalla Man C, Renard E et al (2012) Modular closed-loop control of diabetes. IEEE Trans Biomed Eng 59(11):2986–2999

Peake JM, Tan SJ, Markworth JF, Broadbent JA, Skinner TL, Cameron-Smith D (2014) Metabolic and hormonal responses to isoenergetic high-intensity interval exercise and continuous moderate-intensity exercise. Am J Physiol Endocrinol Metab 307(7):E539–E552

de Pereda D, Romero-Vivo S, Ricarte B, Rossetti P, Ampudia-Blasco FJ, Bondia J (2016) Real-time estimation of plasma insulin concentration from continuous glucose monitor measurements. Comput Methods Biomech Biomed Eng 19(9):934–942

Perfect MM, Patel PG, Scott RE, Wheeler MD, Patel C, Griffin K, Sorensen ST, Goodwin JL, Quan SF (2012) Sleep, glucose, and daytime functioning in youth with type 1 diabetes. Sleep 35(1):81–88

Perkins BA, Riddell MC (2006) Type 1 diabetes and exercise: using the insulin pump to maximum advantage. Can J Diabetes 30(1):72–79

Pettus J, Hirsch I, Edelman S (2013) GLP-1 agonists in type 1 diabetes. Clin Immunol 149(3):317–323

Peyser T, Dassau E, Breton M, Skyler JS (2014) The artificial pancreas: current status and future prospects in the management of diabetes. Ann New York Acad Sci 1311(1):102–123

Phillip M, Battelino T, Atlas E, Kordonouri O, Bratina N, Miller S, Biester T, Avbelj Stefanija M, Muller I, Nimri R et al (2013) Nocturnal glucose control with an artificial pancreas at a diabetes camp. New Engl J Med 368(9):824–833

Pickup J, Keen H (2002) Continuous subcutaneous insulin infusion at 25 years evidence base for the expanding use of insulin pump therapy in type 1 diabetes. Diabetes Care 25(3):593–598

Pleus S, Schmid C, Link M, Zschornack E, Klötzer HM, Haug C, Freckmann G (2013) Performance evaluation of a continuous glucose monitoring system under conditions similar to daily life. J Diabetes Sci Technol 7(4):833–841

Polonsky KS (2012) The past 200 years in diabetes. New Engl J Med 367(14):1332–1340

Pontryagin LS (1987) Mathematical theory of optimal processes. CRC Press

Poolsup N, Suksomboon N, Kyaw AM (2013) Systematic review and meta-analysis of the effectiveness of continuous glucose monitoring (CGM) on glucose control in diabetes. Diabetol Metab Syndr 5(1):1

Poretsky L (2010) Principles of diabetes mellitus, vol 21. Springer

Prime Group for JDRF (2011) Type 1 diabetes, 2010

Puckett WR (1992) Dynamic modelling of diabetes mellitus. University of Wisconsin–Madison

Quon MJ, Cochran C, Taylor SI, Eastman RC (1994) Non-insulin-mediated glucose disappearance in subjects with IDDM: discordance between experimental results and minimal model analysis. Diabetes 43(7):890–896

Rebrin K, Steil GM, van Antwerp WP, Mastrototaro JJ (1999) Subcutaneous glucose predicts plasma glucose independent of insulin: implications for continuous monitoring. Am J Physiol 277(3 Pt 1):E561–E571

Reed K, Lehmann ED (2005) Diabetes website review: www.2aida.org. Diabetes Technol Therap 7(5):741–754

Reifman J, Rajaraman S, Gribok A, Ward WK (2007) Predictive monitoring for improved management of glucose levels. J Diabetes Sci Technol 1(4):478–486

Renard E, Farret A, Kropff J, Bruttomesso D, Messori M, Place J, Visentin R, Calore R, Toffanin C, Di Palma F et al (2016) Day-and-night closed-loop glucose control in patients with type 1 diabetes under free-living conditions: results of a single-arm 1-month experience compared with a previously reported feasibility study of evening and night at home. Diabetes Care 39(7):1151–1160

Report M (2016) FDA advisory panel votes to recommend non-adjunctive use of Dexcom G5 Mobile CGM. Diabetes Technol Therap 18(8):512–516

Rhinehart R (1995) A watchdog for controller performance monitoring. In: American control conference (ACC), vol 3. IEEE, pp 2239–2240

Riazi A, Pickup J, Bradley C (2004) Daily stress and glycaemic control in type 1 diabetes: individual differences in magnitude, direction, and timing of stress-reactivity. Diabetes Res Clin Pract 66(3):237–244

Riddell MC, Zaharieva DP, Yavelberg L, Cinar A, Jamnik VK (2015) Exercise and the development of the artificial pancreas: one of the more difficult series of hurdles. J Diabetes Sci Technol 9(6):1217–1226

Riddell MC, Gallen IW, Smart CE, Taplin CE, Adolfsson P, Lumb AN, Kowalski A, Rabasa-Lhoret R, McCrimmon RJ, Hume C et al (2017) Exercise management in type 1 diabetes: a consensus statement. Lancet Diabetes Endocrinol 5(5):377–390

Riveline JP, Schaepelynck P, Chaillous L, Renard E, Sola-Gazagnes A, Penfornis A, Tubiana-Rufi N, Sulmont V, Catargi B, Lukas C et al (2012) Assessment of patient-led or physician-driven continuous glucose monitoring in patients with poorly controlled type 1 diabetes using basal-bolus insulin regimens a 1-year multicenter study. Diabetes Care 35(5):965–971

Rodbard D (2016) Continuous glucose monitoring: a review of successes, challenges, and opportunities. Diabetes Technol Therap 18(S2):S2–3

Rollo J (1797) An account of two cases of the diabetes mellitus: with remarks, as they arose during the progress of the cure. to which are added, A general view of the nature of the disease and its appropriate treatment, Including observations on some diseases depending on stomach affection; and a detail of the communications received on the subject since the dispersion of the notes on the first case. By John Rollo, MD surgeon-general, Royal Artillery. With the results of the trials of various acids and other substances in the treatment of the Lues Venerea; and some observations on the nature of sugar. By William Cruickshank, Chemist to the ordnance, and a surgeon of artillery. In two volumes. T. Gillet

Romagnoli JA, Palazoglu A (2005) Introduction to process control. CRC Press

Roy A, Parker RS (2006) Dynamic modeling of free fatty acid, glucose, and insulin: an extended "minimal model". Diabetes Technol Therap 8(6):617–626

Roy A, Parker RS (2007) Dynamic modeling of exercise effects on plasma glucose and insulin levels. J Diabetes Sci Technol 1(3):338–347

Russell SJ (2015) Progress of artificial pancreas devices toward clinical use: the first outpatient studies. Curr Opin Endocrinol Diabetes Obes 22(2):106

Russell SJ, El-Khatib FH, Nathan DM, Magyar KL, Jiang J, Damiano ER (2012) Blood glucose control in type 1 diabetes with a bihormonal bionic endocrine pancreas. Diabetes Care 35(11):2148–2155

Russell SJ, El-Khatib FH, Sinha M, Magyar KL, McKeon K, Goergen LG, Balliro C, Hillard MA, Nathan DM, Damiano ER (2014) Outpatient glycemic control with a bionic pancreas in type 1 diabetes. New Engl J Med 371(4):313–325

Russell SJ, Hillard MA, Balliro C, Magyar KL, Selagamsetty R, Sinha M, Grennan K, Mondesir D, Ehklaspour L et al (2016) Day and night glycaemic control with a bionic pancreas versus conventional insulin pump therapy in preadolescent children with type 1 diabetes: a randomised crossover trial. Lancet Diabetes Endocrinol 4(3):233–243

Saboo BD, Talaviya PA (2012) Continuous subcutaneous insulin infusion: practical issues. Indian J Endocrinol Metab 16(Supplement 2):S259

Samadi S, Turksoy K, Hajizadeh I, Feng J, Sevil M, Cinar A (2017) Meal detection and carbohydrate estimation using continuous glucose sensor data. IEEE J Biomed Health Inf 21(3):619–627

Schaepelynck P, Darmon P, Molines L, Jannot-Lamotte M, Treglia C, Raccah D (2011) Advances in pump technology: insulin patch pumps, combined pumps and glucose sensors, and implanted pumps. Diabetes Metab 37:S85–S93

Seborg DE, Mellichamp DA, Edgar TF, Doyle III FJ (2010) Process dynamics and control. Wiley

Senseonics (2017). http://ous.eversensediabetes.com/products/eversense-sensor/

Sevil M, Hajizadeh I, Samadi S, Feng J, Lazaro C, Frantz N, Yu X, Brandt R, Maloney Z, Cinar A (2017) Social and competition stress detection with wristband physiological signals. In: IEEE 14th international conference on wearable and implantable body sensor networks (BSN). IEEE, pp 39–42

Shen Q, Qin SJ, Doniger KJ (2010) Online dropout detection in subcutaneously implanted continuous glucose monitoring. In: American control conference (ACC). IEEE, pp 4373–4378

Sherr JL, Cengiz E, Palerm CC, Clark B, Kurtz N, Roy A, Carria L, Cantwell M, Tamborlane WV, Weinzimer SA (2013) Reduced hypoglycemia and increased time in target using closed-loop insulin delivery during nights with or without antecedent afternoon exercise in type 1 diabetes. Diabetes Care 36(10):2909–2914

Sherr JL, Collazo MP, Cengiz E, Michaud C, Carria L, Steffen AT, Weyman K, Zgorski M, Tichy E, Tamborlane WV et al (2014) Safety of nighttime 2-hour suspension of basal insulin in pump-treated type 1 diabetes even in the absence of low glucose. Diabetes Care 37(3):773–779

Shils M, Olson J, Shike M, Ross A (1998) Fiber and other dietary factors affecting nutrient absorption and metabolism. In: Modern nutrition in health and disease, 9th edn. Baltomore, MD, pp 679–698

Siddiqi S, Boots B, Gordon G (2008) A Constraint generation approach to learning stable linear dynamical systems. Technical report, DTIC document

Signal M, Le Compte A, Harris DL, Weston PJ, Harding JE, Chase JG et al (2012) Using stochastic modelling to identify unusual continuous glucose monitor measurements and behaviour, in newborn infants. Biomed Eng Online 11(1):45

Skladnev VN, Tarnavskii S, McGregor T, Ghevondian N, Gourlay S, Jones TW (2010) Hypoglycemia alarm enhancement using data fusion

Söderström T, Stoica P (1988) System identification. Prentice-Hall, Inc

Sorensen JT (1985) A physiologic model of glucose metabolism in man and its use to design and assess improved insulin therapies for diabetes. PhD thesis, Massachusetts Institute Of Technology

Spaan N, Teplova A, Stam G, Spaan J, Lucas C (2014) Systematic review: continuous intraperitoneal insulin infusion with implantable insulin pumps for diabetes mellitus. Acta Diabetol 51(3):339–351

Srinivasan B, Primus C, Bonvin D, Ricker N (2001) Run-to-run optimization via control of generalized constraints. Control Eng Practice 9(8):911–919

Steil G, Palerm C, Kurtz N, Voskanyan G, Roy A, Paz S, Kandeel F (2011) The effect of insulin feedback on closed loop glucose control. J Clin Endocrinol Metab 96(5):1402–1408

Steil GM (2013) Algorithms for a closed-loop artificial pancreas: the case for proportional-integral-derivative control. J Diabetes Sci Technol 7(6):1621–1631

Steil GM, Rebrin K (2008) Closed loop system for controlling insulin infusion. US Patent 7,354,420

Steil GM, Rebrin K, Darwin C, Hariri F, Saad MF (2006) Feasibility of automating insulin delivery for the treatment of type 1 diabetes. Diabetes 55(12):3344–3350

Stenerson M, Cameron F, Payne SR, Payne SL, Ly TT, Wilson DM, Buckingham BA (2014a) The impact of accelerometer use in exercise-associated hypoglycemia prevention in type 1 diabetes. J Diabetes Sci Technol 9(1):80–85

Stenerson M, Cameron F, Wilson DM, Harris B, Payne S, Bequette BW, Buckingham BA (2014b) The impact of accelerometer and heart rate data on hypoglycemia mitigation in type 1 diabetes. J Diabetes Sci Technol 8(1):64–69

Surwit RS, Schneider MS (1993) Role of stress in the etiology and treatment of diabetes mellitus. Psychosom Med 55(4):380–393

Swan KL, Weinzimer SA, Dziura JD, Steil GM, Voskanyan GR, Steffen AT, Martin ML, Tamborlane WV (2008) Effect of puberty on the pharmacodynamic and pharmacokinetic properties of insulin pump therapy in youth with type 1 diabetes. Diabetes Care 31(1):44–46

Swan KL, Dziura JD, Steil GM, Voskanyan GR, Sikes KA, Steffen AT, Martin ML, Tamborlane WV, Weinzimer SA (2009) Effect of age of infusion site and type of rapid-acting analog on pharmacodynamic parameters of insulin boluses in youth with type 1 diabetes receiving insulin pump therapy. Diabetes Care 32(2):240–244

Taleb N, Emami A, Suppere C, Messier V, Legault L, Ladouceur M, Chiasson JL, Haidar A, Rabasa-Lhoret R (2016) Efficacy of single-hormone and dual-hormone artificial pancreas during continuous and interval exercise in adult patients with type 1 diabetes: randomised controlled crossover trial. Diabetologia 59(12):2561–2571

Taleb N, Haidar A, Messier V, Gingras V, Legault L, Rabasa-Lhoret R (2017) Glucagon in artificial pancreas systems: potential benefits and safety profile of future chronic use. Diabetes Obes Metab 19(1):13–23

Tatara E, Çinar A (2002) An intelligent system for multivariate statistical process monitoring and diagnosis. ISA Trans 41(2):255–270

Thabit H, Tauschmann M, Allen JM, Leelarathna L, Hartnell S, Wilinska ME, Acerini CL, Dellweg S, Benesch C, Heinemann L et al (2015) Home use of an artificial beta cell in type 1 diabetes. New Engl J Med 373(22):2129–2140

Tidelpool (2017). http://tidepool.org

Ting JA, Theodorou E, Schaal S (2007) Learning an outlier-robust Kalman filter. In: ECML. Springer, pp 748–756

Toffanin C, Messori M, Cobelli C, Magni L (2017a) Automatic adaptation of basal therapy for type 1 diabetic patients: a run-to-run approach. Biomed Signal Process Control 31:539–549

Toffanin C, Visentin R, Messori M, Di Palma F, Magni L, Cobelli C (2017b) Towards a run-to-run adaptive artificial pancreas: in silico results. IEEE Trans Biomed Eng

Tsang T, Clarke DW (1988) Generalised predictive control with input constraints. IEE Proc D (Control Theory Appl) 135(6):451–460

Turksoy K, Bayrak ES, Quinn L, Littlejohn E, Cinar A (2013a) Adaptive multivariable closed-loop control of blood glucose concentration in patients with type 1 diabetes. In: American control conference, pp 2905–2910

Turksoy K, Bayrak ES, Quinn L, Littlejohn E, Cinar A (2013b) Multivariable adaptive closed-loop control of an artificial pancreas without meal and activity announcement. Diabetes Technol Therap 15(5):386–400

Turksoy K, Bayrak ES, Quinn L, Littlejohn E, Rollins DK, Cinar A (2013c) Hypoglycemia early alarm systems based on multivariable models. Ind Eng Chem Res 52(35):12,329–12,336

Turksoy K, Bayrak ES, Quinn L, Littlejohn E, Cinar A (2014a) An integrated multivariable artificial pancreas control system. J Diabetes Sci Technol 8(3):498–507

Turksoy K, Quinn L, Littlejohn E, Cinar A (2014b) Multivariable adaptive identification and control for artificial pancreas systems. IEEE Trans Biomed Eng 61(3):883–891

Turksoy K, Paulino TML, Zaharieva DP, Yavelberg L, Jamnik V, Riddell MC, Cinar A (2015) Classification of physical activity information to artificial pancreas control systems in real time. J Diabetes Sci Technol 9(6):1200–1207

Turksoy K, Samadi S, Feng J, Littlejohn E, Quinn L, Cinar A (2016) Meal detection in patients with type 1 diabetes: a new module for the multivariable adaptive artificial pancreas control system. IEEE J Biomed Health Inf 20(1):47–54

Turksoy K, Frantz N, Quinn L, Dumin M, Kilkus J, Hibner B, Cinar A, Littlejohn E (2017a) Automated insulin delivery the light at the end of the tunnel. J Pediatr 186:17–28

Turksoy K, Hajizadeh I, Littlejohn E, Cinar A (2017b) Multivariate statistical monitoring of sensor faults of a multivariable artificial pancreas. In: 20th IFAC world congress. IFAC-PapersOnline 50(1):10998–11004

Turksoy K, Hajizadeh I, Samadi S, Feng J, Sevil M, Park M, Quinn L, Littlejohn E, Cinar A (2017c) Real-time insulin bolusing for unannounced meals with artificial pancreas. Control Eng Pract 59:159–164

Turksoy K, Monforti C, Park M, Griffith G, Quinn L, Cinar A (2017d) Use of wearable sensors and biometric variables in an artificial pancreas system. Sensors 17(3):532

Turksoy K, Roy A, Cinar A (2017e) Real-time model-based fault detection of continuous glucose sensor measurements. IEEE Trans Biomed Eng 64(7):1437–1445

Turksoy K, Littlejohn E, Cinar A (2018) Multimodule, multivariable artificial pancreas for patients with type 1 diabetes. IEEE Control Syst Mag 38(1):105–124. https://doi.org/10.1109/MCS.2017.2766326

Turner SL, Queen TL, Butner J, Wiebe D, Berg CA (2016) Variations in daily sleep quality and type 1 diabetes management in late adolescents. J Pediatr Psychol 41(6):661–669

TypeZeroTechnologies (2017). http://typezero.com

Ündey C, Tatara E, Çınar A (2003) Real-time batch process supervision by integrated knowledge-based systems and multivariate statistical methods. Eng Appl Artif Intell 16(5):555–566

Van Bon AC, Jonker LD, Koebrugge R, Koops R, Hoekstra JB, DeVries JH (2012) Feasibility of a bihormonal closed-loop system to control postexercise and postprandial glucose excursions. J Diabetes Sci Technol 6(5):1114–1122

Vashist SK (2013) Continuous glucose monitoring systems: a review. Diagnostics 3(4):385–412

Vaughn D, Muchmore D (2011) Use of recombinant human hyaluronidase to accelerate rapid insulin analogue absorption: experience with subcutaneous injection and continuous infusion. Endocr Pract 17(6):914–921

Venkatasubramanian V, Rengaswamy R, Yin K, Kavuri SN (2003) A review of process fault detection and diagnosis: part I: quantitative model-based methods. Comput Chem Eng 27(3):293–311

Vicini P, Cobelli C (2001) The iterative two-stage population approach To IVGTT minimal modeling: improved precision with reduced sampling. Am J Physiol Endocrinol Metab 280(1):E179–E186

Walsh J, Roberts R (2006) Pumping insulin, 4th edn. Torrey Pines Press

Walsh J, Roberts R, Bailey T (2010) Guidelines for insulin dosing in continuous subcutaneous insulin infusion using new formulas from a retrospective study of individuals with optimal glucose levels. J Diabetes Sci Technol 4(5):1174–1181

Wan EA, Van Der Merwe R (2000) The unscented Kalman filter for nonlinear estimation. In: The IEEE adaptive systems for signal processing, communications, and control symposium, AS-SPCC. IEEE, pp 153–158

Ward W, Castle J, El Youssef J (2011) Safe glycemic management during closed-loop treatment of type 1 diabetes: the role of glucagon, use of multiple sensors, and compensation for stress hyperglycemia. J Diabetes Sci Technol 5(6):1373–1380

Weber KM, Martin I, Best JD, Alford FP, Boston RC (1989) Alternative method for minimal model analysis of intravenous glucose tolerance data. Am J Physiol Endocrinol Metab 256(4):E524–E535

Weinzimer SA, Steil GM, Swan KL, Dziura J, Kurtz N, Tamborlane WV (2008) Fully automated closed-loop insulin delivery versus semiautomated hybrid control in pediatric patients with type 1 diabetes using an artificial pancreas. Diabetes Care 31(5):934–939

Weissberg-Benchell J, Antisdel-Lomaglio J, Seshadri R (2003) Insulin pump therapy a meta-analysis. Diabetes Care 26(4):1079–1087

Wentholt IM, Hart AA, Hoekstra JB, Devries JH (2007) Relationship between interstitial and blood glucose in type 1 diabetes patients: delay and the push-pull phenomenon revisited. Diabetes Technol Therap 9(2):169–175

WHO Consultation (1999) Definition, diagnosis and classification of diabetes mellitus and its complications, vol 1. World Health Organization

Wiesli P, Schmid C, Kerwer O, Nigg-Koch C, Klaghofer R, Seifert B, Spinas GA, Schwegler K (2005) Acute psychological stress affects glucose concentrations in patients with type 1 diabetes following food intake but not in the fasting state. Diabetes Care 28(8):1910–1915

Wikipedia (2017) History of diabetes. https://en.wikipedia.org/wiki/History_of_diabetes

Willis WD, Diago-Cabezudo JI, Madec-Hily A, Aslam A (2013) Medical resource use, disturbance of daily life and burden of hypoglycemia in insulin-treated patients with diabetes: results from a European online survey. Expert Rev Pharmacoecon Outcomes Res 13(1):123–130

Wong JM, Jenkins DJ (2007) Carbohydrate digestibility and metabolic effects. J Nutr 137(11):2539S–2546S

World Health Organization (1964) WHO expert committee on diabetes mellitus. First report: technical report series 310

World Health Organization (1980) WHO expert committee on diabetes mellitus. Second report: technical report series 646

Xie J, Wang Q (2017) A variable state dimension approach to meal detection and meal size estimation: in silico evaluation through basal-bolus insulin therapy for type 1 diabetes. IEEE Trans Biomed Eng 64:1249–1260

Yeshayahu Y, Mahmud FH (2010) Altered sleep patterns in adolescents with type 1 diabetes: implications for insulin regimen. Diabetes Care 33(11):e142–e142

Zhao C, Fu Y (2015) Statistical analysis based online sensor failure detection for continuous glucose monitoring in type 1 diabetes. Chemom Intell Lab Syst 144:128–137

MIX
Papier aus verantwortungsvollen Quellen
Paper from responsible sources
FSC® C105338

If you have any concerns about our products,
you can contact us on
ProductSafety@springernature.com

In case Publisher is established outside the EU,
the EU authorized representative is:
Springer Nature Customer Service Center GmbH
Europaplatz 3, 69115 Heidelberg, Germany

Printed by Libri Plureos GmbH
in Hamburg, Germany